LULU PIERRE

FOR
BLACK &
BI-RACIAL
HAIR

A PARENT'S GUIDE TO
NATURAL HAIR CARE
FOR GIRLS

A HOW TO GUIDE FOR HEALTHY AND GORGEOUS BLACK HAIR
PLUS AN INTRODUCTION TO NATURAL HAIR STYLES

THE NATURAL HAIR CARE SYSTEM ™
- FREE VIDEO BONUS

Firstly thank you so much for purchasing my book! And as a thank you I would like to offer you a special bonus completely for FREE!

I have an online training program to accompany this book called the NATURAL HAIR CARE SYSTEM ™ which is complete with training videos of all our hair care techniques and a personal hair care regime builder.

I would like to offer you one FREE video module from this course to accompany you reading the book.

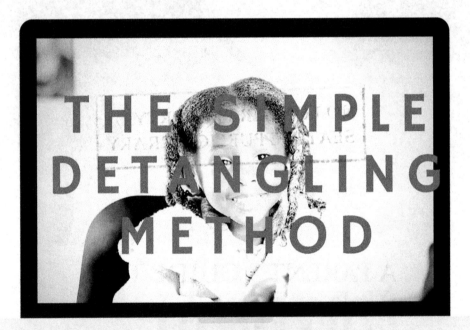

Learn our SIMPLE DETANGLING METHOD with this FREE video training

VISIT: WWW.NATURALHAIRCAREFORGIRLS.COM/AMAZON-BONUS

 WWW.NATURALHAIRCAREFORGIRLS.COM

A PARENT'S GUIDE TO

NATURAL HAIR CARE

FOR GIRLS

LULU PIERRE

A PARENT'S GUIDE TO NATURAL HAIR HAIR FOR GIRLS
A HOW TO GUIDE FOR HEALTHY AND GORGEOUS BLACK HAIR
PLUS AN INTRODUCTION TO NATURAL HAIR STYLES

PUBLISHED IN 2015 BY

BATCH-C PRESS

TABLE OF **CONTENTS**

FROM THE AUTHOR

This was my daughter at 2 years old. She's fully black, has afro-textured hair, and no, those are not hair extensions.

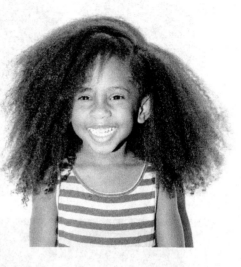

Her hair results were made possible by the techniques I share with you in *A Parent's Guide to Natural Hair Care for Girls.*

After years of dedicated service in my very own hair salon, I heard many mothers complaining of their daughters' kinky, curly or afro hair being dry, thin and appearing not to grow. Turning dry hair into healthy, moisturized hair seemed like an out of reach dream. For them, growing short, damaged hair into long, beautiful hair seemed even more impossible. They didn't know the secrets of cultivating what could very well be healthy, long and beautiful natural hair.

They longed for their daughters to have healthy hair, but were unable to figure out the best practices for reaching that goal. Some opted to give their daughters hair extensions and others opted for chemical relaxers, but the desire for beautiful, natural hair remained.

I've been a relentless student of black hair care and have read all of the best books, blogs and forums on the subject. After attending lots of hair care seminars ,which resulted in me meeting the top-thought leaders in the industry, I created new techniques for optimizing the health and length of kinky, curly and afro-textured hair in children.

I am proud to say that my daughter stands as a testament to what these techniques can do for your daughter.

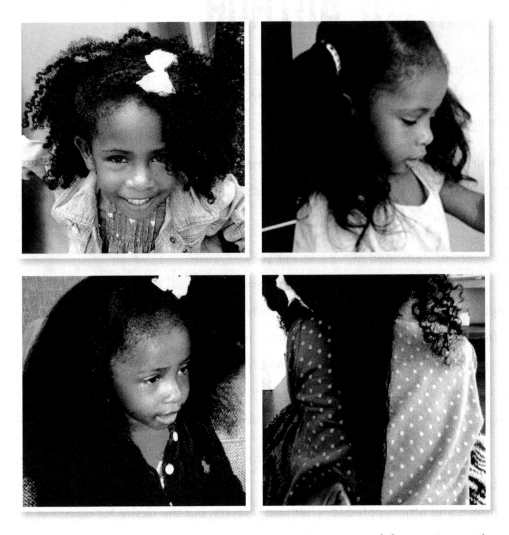

Perhaps you can recall a time when you reached a point of frustration with your daughter's short, dry, brittle or tangling hair?

Before you give up, *A Parent's Guide to Natural Hair Care* for Girls can show you the light.

Written for mothers of *all races* who have a daughter of black or mixed descent with kinky, curly or afro-textured hair, this **step-by-step** guidebook explains in detail and with ease exactly what you need to do to turn it around.

I illustrate for you the pathways to hair salvation.

Maybe your daughter's hair is dry, maybe it's short, maybe it's damaged or maybe you just don't know what hairstyles work best to grow long hair.

This book is a testament of my mission to raise up a whole new generation of black and bi-racial girls with beautiful, long and, most importantly, healthy, natural hair.

This is your opportunity to take action and help your daughter avoid the hair dilemmas often associated with highly textured hair, some of which you may have experienced yourself.

As a professional stylist with over 10 years of experience, I was able to grow my daughter's hair by 12" in only 12 months. In this book, I will walk you through exactly what you need to do to get similar results. I'll also introduce you to natural hairstyling and we will cover the basics of how to plait, cornrow, twist and flat twist for beautiful results.

The techniques and methods in this book have been *proven*.

Together we can take that first step to proving all hair is manageable and beautiful. Each chapter will give you new insights and knowledge of what you need to do. Take control of your daughter's hair, right now, and help her grow beautiful, natural hair today!

Lulu Pierre

CHAPTER 1 INTRODUCTION

WHY THE BOOK?

Well, let me take the time to formally introduce myself! My name is Lulu Pierre and my daughter's name is Bae Rose. I wrote this book to help kids like Bae avoid the confidence issues I faced as a child.

Hair can impact the type of person we become, shaping our style and even our personality. This becomes problematic when you begin to have a power struggle with your hair. As a child, I had a horribly negative relationship with my own hair. In my mind, it never really seemed to grow the way I wanted. I thought it was short and ugly. As you can imagine, my self-image and in turn my self-esteem were always negative.

Speaking with others, I have found that it is an all too common experience to be at war with the natural locks of kinky, curly or afro hair. This inability to make peace with what sits at the crown of our heads often translates into a lifetime of headache.

I want this book to positively impact and change the relationship between a young girl and her curls.

Rather than each school portrait capturing a lost battle with hair products and improper styling, I want this book to empower parents to be able to take control and bring out the true beauty in their daughters kinky, curly and afro locks. Beauty that breeds confidence, and confidence that beams throughout their childhood and coming of age—so that when they grow up, they not only know how to tend to their hair, but can also tend to that of the next generation.

This book is the authoritative guide on how to care for young girls' kinky, curly and afro-textured hair, be she black or bi-racial. My aim is to empower and equip every mother who reads this book with the ability to beautify her daughter's natural hair.

WHY NOW?

I think now is the perfect time for such a book.

It really feels like the natural hair movement is gathering momentum, and I'm really encouraged by it. It seems like more and more women are getting to grips with their natural kinky, curly or afro hair, understanding it and growing it to unfathomed lengths. As a black, afro-haired woman myself, it's a beautiful and an encouraging sight to behold.

It seems like everywhere I turn online, I see women with long and healthy natural hair sharing their stories and advice. You see so many of them that it almost gives the impression that all curly-haired women have got their hair game on point.

But in real life and away from the world wide web, You Tube and social media, there seems to be a different reality.

There are still plenty of curly and afro-haired women out there who are daunted by the idea of caring for their natural tresses, and not only have they not come to grips with their own hair, they have not come to grips with caring for their daughters' hair, either.

I can admit that I myself was daunted by the prospect.

When I was pregnant, I wondered if I would be able to look after my daughter's hair properly. Would it be short, dry and brittle, just as mine had been as a child?

I'd worn extensions for so long that I was completely out of touch with my natural hair. I never understood it, embraced it or really took good care of it.

I found myself presented with two choices: I could either do nothing and hope for the best, or I could become a student of natural black hair and learn how to take care of it properly.

And it's the results of my decision to become a student of natural black hair that I present to you in this book.

WHAT THIS BOOK COVERS

It's with absolute pride that I can boldly say that this book is your ultimate guide to caring for your daughter's natural hair. You will learn the best hair care practices for beautiful, healthy, natural hair, no matter the texture.

We will cover some hair science along with practical theory, with detailed instructions for you to follow. We will also cover the basics of natural hair styling, which includes plaiting, twisting and cornrowing.

WHAT THIS BOOK DOESN'T COVER

Although we do cover the basics of natural hair styling, this isn't a traditional hairstyling book where you will learn lots of intricate styles. Rather, my focus is on hair health, because I believe that is the first objective.

My ethos is that any great style starts with a great foundation, and that foundation is healthy hair.

MY FOCUS

My focus in this book is babies and young children, and the purpose of this is two-fold. The first purpose is practical: we need to understand textured hair and what it needs to thrive. The second purpose is personal: I want to help young girls develop a positive self-image and a positive view of their hair and themselves.

Together we can avoid the creation of a typical horrible hair relationship and turn it into a happy one. This book is my antidote to the qualms and quarrels of having kinky, curly or afro-textured hair.

Seeing a comb should not send your daughter into hiding. Hair washday should not turn into an argument. Our daughters should fall in love with their hair through to adulthood, starting today.

You could call this the natural movement for kids!

CHAPTER 2 THE GOAL OF HAIR CARE

WHAT IS THIS ALL ABOUT, LU?

The first thing we need to understand, before we go any further, is what this is all about, and what it is all for. We need to understand the ultimate goal.

BEGIN WITH THE END IN MIND

I always believe when embarking on a new task or challenge that one must begin with the end goal in mind, and keep it in mind. It's important to not only know what the goal is, but also to design a practical approach for reaching that goal. I see hair care no differently. We need to clearly understand our objectives when caring for our girls' hair.

What is it we want, and why do we want it?

OUR ULTIMATE GOAL

Our ultimate goal for our daughters is for them to have healthy and beautiful hair.

Healthy hair isn't dependent on length, hair type or texture, but can be described as:

- Hair that is **strong** and resilient to breakage.
- Hair that is **moisturized** and retains an appropriate moisture level.
- Hair that has **elasticity** and can be stretched considerably without snapping.
- Hair that is **free from damage** or **breakage**, including split ends, bald, thin or weak spots.

Hair that fits the above description can be described as being in 'good condition,' whereas hair that does not, can be described as being in 'bad condition' or 'unhealthy'.

Some people may include hair shine and softness into the above definition, but I don't think these apply when dealing with textured hair because they are often dictated by curl patterns, and as such are not direct indicators of health.

Shine and sheen are simply determined by how well the hair reflects light. Some hair textures can be very healthy, but have low sheen because they do not reflect light well. For example, straight hair often has a lot more shine than curly hair. Similarly, some textures of hair are naturally softer than others, but that doesn't mean they are healthier, and that's why I didn't include them.

Healthy hair is obtained through consistent healthy hair care practices *over time*. Our end hair goal, therefore, is our motivator to stay on the journey, even if we are faced with challenges.

WHAT ARE HEALTHY HAIR CARE PRACTICES?

Simply put, healthy hair care practices are the methods we use to either maintain or *improve* the condition of the hair.

We will only ever maintain the hair's present condition if it is healthy hair as described above. We will improve the hair's condition if it shows any signs of weakness, dryness, breakage or damage.

We absolutely never want to adopt hair care practices that cause the health of the hair to decline, because this is going completely against our objective.

UNHEALTHY HAIR

Unhealthy hair can be described as hair that is weak, dry, brittle, damaged or broken. If anything we are doing to the hair causes it to be unhealthy, we need to stop and evaluate what is going wrong.

We need to be aware that ***unhealthy hair happens slowly*** and it could be that we are adopting unhealthy hair care practices or bad products without having a clue. In this book, I will present only the practices and products needed to obtain healthy hair.

Unhealthy hair is our enemy and we need systems in place so we can avoid it. Once hair is severely damaged, it cannot be repaired and will have to be cut, which we want to avoid entirely!

HEALTHY HAIR IS POSSIBLE

It is possible for all hair types and textures to be healthy. Many people with textured hair seem to dismiss any notion of healthy hair for themselves. This defeatist attitude dominates many clients and individuals I have observed, leading to a generally poor outlook.

There are some people who genuinely believe that black hair can't be healthy or it can't grow, or that it is intrinsically 'bad' hair. Before we move on, we need to dispel some prevailing and damaging myths.

CHAPTER 3 HAIR MYTHS DEBUNKED

As we enter the journey of healthy hair with our daughters, it's important we have the knowledge to dispel some common misconceptions that surround black and bi-racial hair.

In order to build up a healthy routine, a foundation of not only practices, but also one of information, is important. In order to truly appreciate highly textured hair, understanding its nature and debunking myths surrounding it will not only improve attitudes towards it, but will also empower us as mothers to take control and help our daughters build a positive self-image.

As a salon owner, I encountered many common misconceptions that you may have also been exposed to yourself. I admit that I myself held some of these beliefs, and they did hinder my personal hair journey. There were times when I lost hope and let go of any real goals for my hair.

I believed healthy, beautiful hair wasn't possible for people like me. I had to unlearn a lot of this misinformation before I was able to fully commit to my daughter having healthy hair. Hence, you may have to prepare yourself for deconstructing that which you have held as fact all this time.

By debunking these myths and presenting you with the facts, I hope to renew your mind so you are fully able to believe and commit to the process.

(MYTH NUMBER ONE)
BLACK HAIR IS UGLY, UNMANAGEABLE AND UNDESIRABLE
Firstly, we need to understand that not all black people feel this way, but some do and it's often an internalized value held consciously or sub-consciously. I can confess that I held it myself.

It's more something that needs to be un-learnt, rather than consciously learnt, because for some it can almost seem like a normal and logical way of thinking and often starts from early childhood.

It's important for one to dispel this rationale, because it imposes self-limitation. In this context, if a mother believes her daughter's hair can only be ugly, unmanageable and undesirable, and she acts on what she believes, she will achieve very little. But if she *believes* her daughter's hair has the capability to be beautiful, healthy and long, she will act on that and achieve what the unbelieving mother won't.

The natural hair movement is so significant to black women, because it signifies a mental shift in their perception of their hair and, in turn, themselves. It seems we are getting to a place where the versatility and beauty of kinky, curly and afro hair is being fully appreciated.

I agree with Patricia 'Deecoily' Gaines of the blog 'Nappyturality', who counters the idea of being ugly, unmanageable and undesirable black hair with the idea that black hair is in fact *"underestimated, undervalued and unloved."*

To understand more about why black women often see their hair so negatively, we have to go back in time. We need to understand the negative effects slavery had on perceptions of black hair on a global scale.

So here's a very brief and simplified overview.

Back in Africa, before slavery reached the western shores, African tribes would style their hair into intricate and elaborate styles. The styles were symbolic, and tribeswomen would spend hours and sometimes days grooming each other to achieve unique looks. They had pride in their hair, as their hairstyles displayed social status and tribal identity.

With the advent of slavery, tribes were displaced and taken to new lands, but were left with no real way to care for their natural hair. African languages, cultures and grooming traditions disappeared and slaves were no longer allowed to maintain traditional hairstyles. Sometimes female slaves had their heads shaved, which as a result cut out their connection to themselves, their past and their sense of self.

To further this distancing of the self, European standards of beauty (light skin, straight hair, fine features) were in turn pushed onto slaves as desirable, and slaves with straighter, less afro-textured hair and lighter skin were sold for higher prices at auction.

As a result, many blacks internalised the idea that the straighter the hair, the better, and the more afro-textured, the worse. Afro hair was seen by many to be of *less value* or 'bad hair' and less attractive than straighter hair, which was deemed to be 'good hair.' The idea of afro hair being inferior was internalised by many.

As one can image, the implications of something as material as hair has left a heavy burden upon today's social values of beauty. These ideas of afro-textured hair being less desirable still exist today, consciously and sub-consciously. This mentality ran so deeply that even post-slavery, 'good hair' became a requirement for entry into certain social circles, jobs, schools and churches. It's a sensitive issue that I can only touch upon here, but I can say that it caused a great many to harbour feelings of inferiority in relation to their hair.

Sadly, this mentality is still alive today, and as evidence of this, I'm sure we have all heard someone use the term when describing another person, saying, for example, "that girl's got *good hair*."

I'm sure if some of us were to sit and quietly reflect, we would be able to see how this mentality has affected us personally. I know I struggled with feelings of ugliness because of it, especially during my teenage years, as I was not one with so-called 'good' hair.

But I'd like to dispel this as a myth, because it was formed synthetically. Black women took such great pride in their hair prior to slavery; they understood it and saw it as a thing of beauty.

It's important that we see all hair types as something of beauty and try to un-learn the hair grading system that seems so entrenched. If we don't, it may obstruct our hair care efforts going forwards.

We do not want to pass this mentality onto a new generation, who should grasp their full potential and utilize it. In order for our hair to not be damaged, our ideas and perceptions should not begin to be damaged in childhood.

Your daughter will need to hear from **you** that her hair is beautiful and something of value. Reinforcing these values will help her faith grow in not only her potential, but in her self-worth as well.

(MYTH NUMBER 2)

BLACK HAIR DOESN'T GROW! (OR GROWS *REALLY* SLOWLY)

This is largely a myth. I say largely because there are some diagnosable medical conditions that can affect hair growth, but in the absence of these, it's another one that has to go.

I can't tell you the number of times I've heard this one, and people sincerely believe it. My salon clients would tell me their 'hair doesn't grow' every single day.

I even recall my own father saying that my hair 'didn't grow'. I believed him. Indeed, my hair did not get long. But was it really a case of growth, or of care? Does black hair sometimes not grow?

To get to the truth, we need to get the facts.

According to Audrey Davis-Sivasothy, in her amazing book *The Science of Black Hair:*

"All hair grows at the rate of ¼ - ½ an inch per month."

And the website Wikipedia states:

*"The rate or speed of hair growth is about 1.25 centimetres or 0.5 inches per month, or about 15 centimetres or **6 inches per year.**"*

This is *irrespective of race*. Yes, these are average growth rates, so some of us will experience more or less, but you get the point.

I'm guessing that by now some of you may be a little confused as to why it seems black people have shorter hair, or why it seems not to grow, but that has more to do with other factors and not the speed of growth.

There are two factors at play here that either keep black hair short or appearing short: breakage and shrinkage.

BREAKAGE AS A CAUSE OF SHORT HAIR

The cold hard truth of the matter is this. **Hair breakage is the number one enemy of black hair.** It is a key contributor to perpetually short hair: that is, hair that *appears* to not grow.

The issue here is with length retention. Length retention is basically the state when hair strands don't break as they grow, so new growth can be seen.

Let me give you an example. If a person's hair grows ½" per month, yet breaks ½" per month, the hair will appear to NOT GROW. This person will suffer from what is termed short hair syndrome.

SHORT HAIR SYNDROME

Short hair syndrome occurs as a result of hair breaking as fast as it grows, and this occurs in hair that is dry, damaged and brittle. So the key to overcoming it is to raise health levels in the hair so it doesn't break, and therefore length can be realized.

Looking back at our example, if a person's hair grows 1/2" a month and does not break at all, in one year, that person's hair will be 6" longer.

BREAKAGE IS SO COMMON

As a child, I recall constantly seeing broken hairs after combing, washing or blow-drying. I thought this was normal, as many people do, because it happens almost every time they style or manage their hair. Some even see it as part of the territory of having black hair. But the actual truth is, it's not normal, nor is it tolerable. It should be addressed immediately.

To overcome short hair syndrome, the first step is to **eradicate breakage** by taking steps to make sure the hair is healthy. Stopping breakage not only retains the original length of the hair, but it ensures healthy growth. Then, and only then, can we see it get longer.

SHRINKAGE AS A CAUSE OF SHORT HAIR

Another reason black hair can be seen as short is in part due to shrinkage. Love it or hate it, shrinkage does come with the territory of having highly textured hair, but it doesn't actually mean the hair is short; rather, it *appears* short.

It has been estimated that afro hair can shrink up to 75% of its stretched length in its shrunken state. That's a whole lot of length, and to put that into context, imagine someone with 10" hair stretched. Those 10", when shrunk, can appear to be as short as 2.5"!

Shrunk hair is the default setting for natural afro hair. If it has been stretched and gets wet or is washed, it will revert and shrinkage will set in! But shrinkage should not be automatically deemed as a bad thing. Rather, it is a part of the unique package that makes afro hair what it is.

LENGTH CHECK AS A WAY TO SEE GROWTH

Hair length in afro hair can be revealed when the hair is stretched. A common way to do this is through blow-drying or flat ironing. Often naturals will straighten their hair to do a 'length check' to check in on their progress.

Don't assume just because someone appears to have short hair that this is the case. All too often shrinkage is hiding major length!

(MYTH NUMBER 3)

ONLY MIXED PEOPLE CAN GROW REALLY LONG HAIR

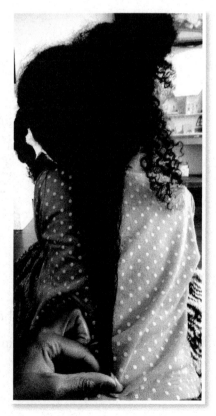

In my experience, this one is very pervasive and coincides with the all too common myth that black hair is inferior. For many, it's a completely normal and logical way to think.

I've been following healthy hair practices with my daughter since she was born, and now at 3 years old her hair is close to waist length when stretched. Her hair is very long, and time and time again I am asked if she is mixed with anything other than black. She isn't.

Some people just can't comprehend that a fully black person can have hair that long. They even try to convince me, her very own mother, that my daughter must be mixed! It's unfortunate how deeply embedded this mentality has been weaved into the logic of some.

Looking at the topic through a scientific lens, we've established that on average hair grows about 6" per year. But what we need to know next, in order to understand its length potential, is to understand the *length of time* it can grow for.

To understand this we need to learn about the human hair growth cycle.

THE HUMAN HAIR GROWTH CYCLE

The hair growth cycle consists of 3 distinct phases, the anagen (growth) phase, the catagen (rest) phase and the telegen (shed) phase.

LET'S LOOK IN A BIT MORE DETAIL.

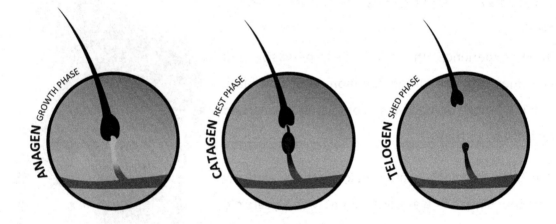

ANAGEN/GROWTH PHASE

The growth phase is a stage in the hair cycle where a hair is consistently growing. At any one time an average of 88% of individual hairs on our head are in the anagen phase.

CATAGEN/REST PHASE

At the end of the anagen phase, the follicle will go into a rest phase, where it will stop growing. This period lasts about 2 weeks.

TELEGEN/SHED PHASE

This is the final stage in the growth journey, and it's the point at which resting hair begins to shed. The follicle then remains inactive for about 3 months, until the whole process begins again.

It's important to note that each hair on our head operates independently and goes through the cycle at different times; otherwise we would go completely bald in the shed phase! Instead, an adult will normally shed between 80–100 hairs a day.

TERMINAL LENGTH

Terminal length can be described as the maximum length hair can grow to, and it's determined by genetics.

So by now some of you may be thinking that maybe black people are genetically predisposed to having shorter hair. But this is not the case.

The human hair growth phase can last anywhere between 2–7 years, regardless of race.

Putting this into more context: if a person's hair grows at the average rate of 6" per year, and their growth cycle is the shortest at 2 years, then they can grow at least 12" of hair. Of course, this is oversimplified, because it doesn't take into account factors such as breakage or haircuts, but hopefully it illustrates the point of hair growth potential.

The growth phase can be anything from 2–7 years, so my above example is for someone with the shortest phase. Some people have growth phases of up to 7 years and can grow seriously long hair.

AT LEAST 12" INCHES

It's a myth to think that black people cannot grow long hair! I consider 12" to be a decent length myself, and the good news is that it should be the bare minimum that is achievable for anyone, regardless of race.

NO MORE EXCUSES

It's important for us as mums to get our heads around this one, but I will actually take it one step further. It's important to learn the facts, accept them and take responsibility, and not use excuses to pardon yourself from not trying with your daughter's hair.

If you have a young child, then you are the caregiver. If for any reason the hair seems to be suffering, then *you* will need to stop, pay attention and figure out what is going wrong so you can correct it. Strong talk, I know, but I say it with love!

(MYTH NUMBER 4)

GREASE AND OIL CAN MOISTURIZE THE HAIR

I don't know about you, but growing up for me seemed to be all about hair grease.

Grease was pretty much the only product that was applied to my hair apart from shampoo. My mum would use it all over my hair in order to 'moisturize' it, and it appeared to do the trick. Once applied, my hair didn't look dry and even had lots of shine. But was it really moisturized? Let's again look to some facts.

GREASE CAN'T PENETRATE INTO THE HAIR SHAFT

For hair to be moisturized, it needs to receive hydration inside the hair shaft.

Grease can't do this.

Firstly, grease can't offer hair hydration; only water can do this. And secondly its molecules are often too big to penetrate inside the hair shaft.

What ends up occurring is that grease gives the appearance of moisturized hair without the hair actually receiving any moisture.

I know from my personal experience my hair was chronically dry and the grease my mum applied did nothing to hydrate it, which is why it broke so much and I suffered from short hair syndrome.

I believe this myth is particularly damaging as it can contribute to locking us into short hair syndrome, which is what happened to me.

Let me give an example.

THE GREASE TRAP

A child has dry hair, and to combat this, the mum uses grease to 'moisturize' it.

The grease does nothing and delivers zero moisture, but it does leave the hair shiny, making it look moisturized.

Over time, the hair will look dry again, so more grease is applied to 'moisturize' it.

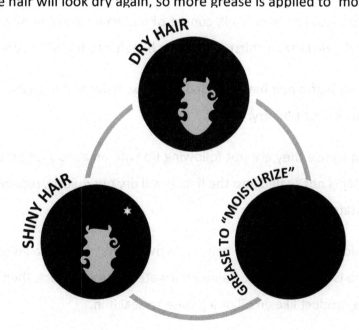

And so the cycle repeats, with the hair never getting any of the crucial moisture it needs. The result is dry and brittle hair that is prone to breaking.

I think this is particularly dangerous because:

1) The mum thinks she is doing the right thing and as a result may blame the breakage on the child's hair.

2) The child may internalize that she has 'bad' hair, because even though she sees her mum looking after it, it still doesn't grow and breaks all the time.

3) The hair will actually get drier because grease is an occlusive agent. This basically means that not only does it lock and seal dryness into the hair, it also creates an external barrier and stops any moisture from entering in.

These three reasons make grease a triple threat to dry hair.

WATER IS THE ANSWER

The best ingredient to moisturize dry hair is water.

Water-based products, or water itself, consist of molecules small enough to penetrate the hair shaft and deliver their thirst-quenching benefits to the hairs core.

Even so, people with afro hair have avoided using excessive water on their hair because they think it makes their hair dry.

But that's only because they are not following up with an adequate product to seal in the water. If water is not sealed into the hair, it will dry out quickly, returning the hair to its original dry state.

You see, water does not stay in the hair on its own; it has to be sealed or locked in. So what we must do is moisturize the hair with a water-based product, then use a heavier, non-penetrating product like an oil or a grease to seal it in.

Nevertheless, we will go into this in more detail later in the book—don't you worry!

It is not that grease has to be avoided like the plague. It can actually work in some circumstances, but it's important to know when to apply it and for what purpose.

(MYTH NUMBER 5)

LOOKING AFTER BLACK HAIR TAKES AGES (AND I DON'T HAVE THE TIME OR ENERGY)

Okay, so I can't completely dispel this one, but I can shed some light on it and this one is all about perspective.

As humans, we instinctively spend time on the things that are important to us, and if something is significant enough, we will *make* the time.

I see hair care in this way. I think the traditional view of maintaining black hair as some sort of chore stems from the erroneous thinking that black hair is unmanageable and provides no one a positive experience. I think the way to overcome this rationale is to change perspective and take a more positive mental approach.

I talked about the goal of hair care in Chapter 2, and I think it's important to focus on achieving healthy hair above all else and work towards that so we stay motivated and focused.

MAKE HAIR TIME ENJOYABLE FOR YOUR DAUGHTER

If you are doing a child's hair, then a major reason it can be an energy drainer is if the child hates having it done.

When a child doesn't like having their hair done, they may cry, squirm and move about a lot. This slows progress and is really tiresome. I can remember not liking hair time when I was a child. It was boring. I could think of 100 things I would rather do than get my hair done!

The best way to overcome this is to make it more interesting. You can do this by involving your daughter, explaining to her what is going on and maybe even getting her to help! Of course, treats are always good incentives.

But the best time to do a child's hair is when they are engrossed in something else. Be it a book, a puzzle or a film, the aim is for them to be totally occupied with something else so you can get on with the job at hand!

IT'S ALL IN THE ATTITUDE

Although I can't deny that yes, okay, sometimes doing a child's hair will take time, it's how you see it that will make all the difference.

I have spoken to some mums who have said that they don't have time to look after their daughters' hair, but I think what they are really saying is "listen, I don't believe black hair deserves the time, I don't believe it will grow anyways, and I don't have the time to wait and wonder."

The myths I'm talking about often affect attitudes and mental approaches to black hair care. That's why it's crucially important to get the facts and be empowered so attitudes can be renewed!

Now that we have dispelled the common myths, let us get into some hard facts about your daughter's hair and what it needs to thrive.

CHAPTER 4 HAIR SCIENCE

It's important, before we move onto the theory of what you need to do to obtain healthy hair, for you to understand *why* you need to do it. This comes from you understanding more about the science of hair itself.

Before I really took time to understand hair science myself, I would hit the same brick wall again and again in my hair journey. I never seemed to grow my hair beyond a certain length without my hair breaking. I couldn't for the life of me figure out what was going on. I knew I had a problem, but I didn't know what it was and definitely didn't know how to solve it.

Enter hair science.

After understanding more about highly textured hair and its unique characteristics, I was able to overcome my hair issues and also avoid similar issues with my daughter. Hopefully so will you.

WHAT IS HAIR, ANYWAY?

Hair is primarily composed of a protein called keratin and grows through the dermis (skin) from follicles beneath the scalp.

It has two parts to it: the root (the part beneath the skin at the base of the follicle) and the shaft (the part you can touch and style).

The base of the root is known as the hair bulb, which is where the hair receives nutrients from the blood stream and where new hair cells are created.

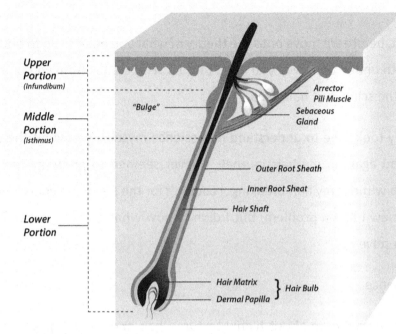

Upper Portion (Infundibum)

Middle Portion (Isthmus)

Lower Portion

"Bulge"

Arrector Pili Muscle

Sebaceous Gland

Outer Root Sheath

Inner Root Sheat

Hair Shaft

Hair Matrix
Dermal Papilla
} Hair Bulb

DEAD OR ALIVE?

There is a lot of misconception out there on this one. You sometimes hear people talking about trimming dead hair or hair looking dead. This is only half of the truth. The hair you can see is dead, but the hair beneath the skin is actually alive. In fact, this is where hair cells regenerate.

Once hair has passed through the follicle and grows out as a strand, the cells within it die and are just a collection of interwoven, protein-rich fibres with no biochemical activity. All the hair we can see on our body contains these dead cells.

HOW DOES IT GROW?

The hair bulb (the base of the follicle) can be described as a structure of actively growing cells that are constantly dividing.

When this happens, the existing older cells are pushed outwards and harden. This, in turn, lengthens the strand and contributes to hair growth.

The process by which the hair passes from the follicle and through the skin is called keratinization, which is essentially where the hair cells die, lose their nucleus, harden and are filled with proteins.

THE STRUCTURE OF HAIR

If we were to dissect a strand of hair, we would see that it's made up of 3 distinct layers: the cuticle, cortex and medulla.

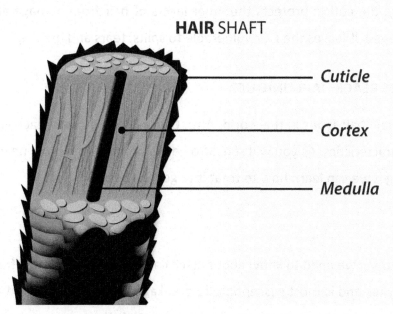

HAIR SHAFT

Cuticle

Cortex

Medulla

THE MEDULLA

This is the innermost part of the hair shaft and is constructed of transparent cells and air spaces. It's only present in large, thick and grey/white hair. Scientists are uncertain as to its exact function.

THE CORTEX

This is the middle layer of the hair strand, between the medulla and cuticle, and forms the main bulk of the hair. It also contains a majority of the hair's pigment melanin. It primarily consists of long keratin filaments held together by disulphide and hydrogen bonds. The health of the cortex depends heavily on the integrity of the hair's cuticle.

THE CUTICLE

The cuticle is the protective outer layer of hair and consists of overlapping cells similar in pattern to fish scales, which face downwards towards the ends of the hair. These cells control the amount of water in and out of the cortex and determine the hair's porosity. When healthy, the cuticle protects the inner layers of hair from damage and gives it shine. If damaged, it leaves the hair vulnerable to splits, tears and breakage.

WHAT MAKES BLACK HAIR UNIQUE?

There are 3 main hair types in the world: Afro, Caucasian and Asian, each with unique traits and characteristics. As you will see, afro hair is probably the most unique, but by understanding it we can learn how to treat it to get the best out of it!

STRENGTH

The very first thing we need to know about black hair is that it is the most fragile of the 3 main hair types and is most susceptible to breakage. Studies have found the tensile strength in afro hair to be the weakest. Tensile strength is the force required to pull on an item in order for it to snap.

Black hair is the weakest and breaks the easiest under pressure, which is not good news as curly hair needs strength to be able to withstand the pressure that comes from combing or detangling.

HAIR STRAND SHAPE

On top of black hair being weak, the unique shape of the strands makes them even *more* susceptible to breakage.

If we look at a cross section of hair from each type, we will see that Asian and Caucasian hair is round in shape, whilst afro hair is oval.

SHAPE OF THE **HAIR**

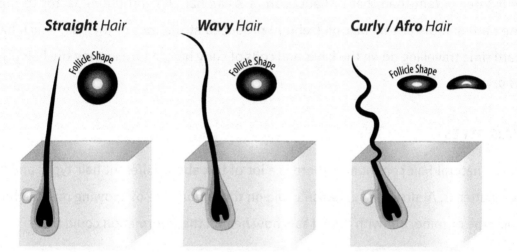

As a result of their oval shape, afro strands are often tightly curled, can have random reversal in direction and have uneven thickness in each strand.

Where an individual strand is at is thinnest, it is also at its weakest. In textured hair, this is most likely to occur where it is needed most: right at the point of a kink or curl.

DENSITY

We often think of kinky and curly hair being thicker or denser than other hair types, but actually it's the least dense of all the hair types. The way the hair curls and coils is what gives it the appearance of thick hair.

Hair density is determined by the number of follicles on the scalp.

Studies by Franbourg et al. found the average density of afro-textured hair to be approximately 190 hairs per square centimetre. This was significantly lower than that of Caucasian hair, which, on average, has approximately 227 hairs per square centimetre.

MOISTURE CONTENT

The same study also found that afro hair is the driest of all hair types, as it has less moisture content than that of Caucasian or Asian hair. A contributing factor to this is the natural moisturizing hair oil (sebum) produced at the root of the hair, which has a hard time travelling down the kinks and coils of curly hair, in turn leaving the hair prone to dryness.

HAIR TYPES

In the natural hair community, there is a lot of talk about different hair types and hair curl patterns. At first glance, I wasn't sold on the importance of knowing my daughter's hair type or mine, but with time, I saw how helpful this information could be.

THE BENEFIT OF KNOWING YOUR HAIR TYPE

The main advantage of knowing your hair type is the ability to diagnose potential problems and issues associated with it.

I, for example, have Type 4 (kinky, afro-textured hair) hair. For a long time, I struggled with severe breakage. After searching for the common problems associated with my hair type, I was able to find a solution that helped me dramatically reduce my breakage. Hair problems and solutions can often be broken down by hair type, which is advantageous.

THE ANDRE WALKER SYSTEM

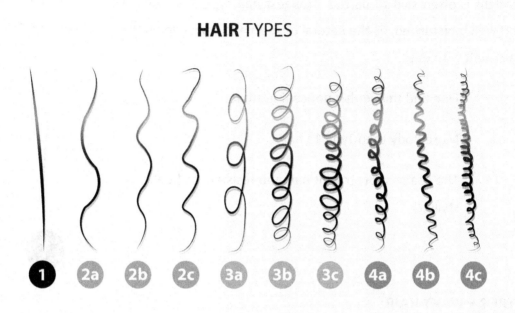

HAIR TYPES

Andre Walker made popular a hair typing system widely used in the natural hair community and identified 4 hair types with 3 possible sub-types.

Most women and girls with curly or afro-textured hair will likely have at least 2 different textures of hair. Many curly-haired individuals find the curls around the perimeter of their head to be looser, while those in the middle and crown can be tighter. Generally, there won't be a great variation in the types of curls, but rather their diameter, making them looser or tighter.

It's important to note that depending on your daughter's age, she may still be developing her established hair texture, so her hair type is subject to change until she gets to around 3–4 years of age, but below is a brief overview.

TYPE 1 – STRAIGHT HAIR

Straight is often said to be the strongest hair type. It's resilient and well moisturized, as the natural oil is able to travel down the hair shaft with ease.

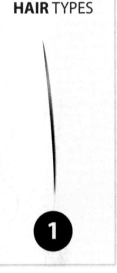

HAIR TYPES

1a – Fine and thin with a noticeable shine.

1b – More body than Type 1a hair.

1c – The coarsest of straight hair and resistant to heat styling.

TYPE 2 – WAVY HAIR

Wavy hair usually isn't overly oily or dry. It's generally thought of as the middle ground between straight and curly hair. It has slightly less natural shine than straight hair.

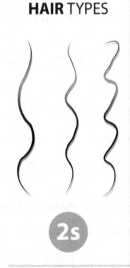

HAIR TYPES

2a – Fine and thin. Easy to curl and straighten.

2b – Tends to have waves that adhere to the shape of the head.

2c – Frizzy waves that are fairly coarse and with less shine.

TYPE 3 – CURLY HAIR

Curls in this rage typically have an 'S' shape when stretched. The cuticle doesn't lay flat in curly hair, so this type will have noticeably less shine than Types 1 and 2 hair.

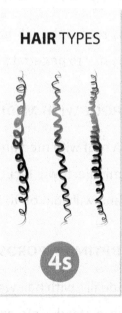

HAIR TYPES

3s

3a – Shiny and loose curls.

3b – Tighter, bouncy curls, spiral-shaped.

3c – Tight spiral curls that look like corkscrews.

TYPE 4 – KINKY HAIR

Commonly referred to as afro hair, this type is comprised of tight curls or 'coils', as they are commonly called. It is extremely fragile and can be the driest hair type with the least shine. Hair strands are often fine.

HAIR TYPES

4s

4a – Coils that have an 'S' shape when stretched. Some curl definition.

4b – Less definition. Coils appear to have a 'Z' pattern as the hair bends at sharp angles.

4c – Very similar to 4b, but will have no curl definition as coils will not clump together.

If your daughter has afro-textured hair, then it's highly likely that she will have hair that falls into the Types 3 and 4 range, and as you now know, these hair types are in fact the weakest and require the most care and attention in order to thrive.

Although hair typing can be helpful in understanding more about black hair, unfortunately it doesn't tell the whole story. To understand further, we need to learn about hair porosity and hair strand thickness.

HAIR POROSITY: WHAT IS IT?

Simply put, hair porosity is the amount of water the hair can absorb and retain. A good way to understand it is to think of tiles on a roof.

ROOF WITH LOW POROSITY

Roofs with low porosity will have tiles that lay completely flat. It will be extremely difficult for water to penetrate it, and if any does, it will be difficult for it to escape.

ROOF WITH HIGH POROSITY

A roof with high porosity will have tiles that are raised; it will be extremely easy for water to penetrate it and just as easy for it to escape.

ROOF WITH MEDIUM POROSITY

A roof with medium porosity will have tiles that are neither raised nor flat, but sit in the middle. It will let in more water than low porosity hair and less than high porosity hair, and will hold on to it for a reasonable amount of time.

OPTIMUM POROSITY

Ideally, with hair we want to have medium porosity because we want it to absorb water at a steady rate and retain it for a reasonable amount of time. Low porosity hair is not ideal because its inability to absorb water will leave the hair prone to dryness and breakage. Similarly, high porosity is not ideal, because although it is able to absorb water well, it loses it just as fast, and this also leaves the hair prone to dryness and breakage.

Understanding hair porosity is a critical component in any hair regime, because it will affect your approach towards having healthy, moisturized hair. We will learn how to test for porosity and choose appropriate products in the 'How to select products' chapter.

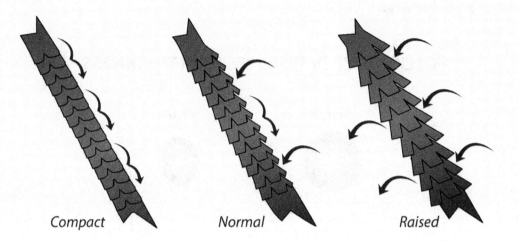

Compact   *Normal*   *Raised*

Porosity
Compact Cuticle (Low Porosity)
Normal ; Raised Cuticle (High Porosity)

HAIR STRAND THICKNESS

Another component we need to understand in the quest for healthy hair is the thickness of the hair strands themselves. When we identify whether our daughters' hair strands are thick or thin, it helps us understand more about the needs of the hair.

Textured hair usually falls into 2 categories:

THIN/SKINNY

Skinny strands are very common in Type 4 hair. They have a small circumference, a small internal area and a smaller cuticle surface area than fatter strands, which makes them delicate and prone to breakage.

THICK/FATTER

Fatter strands have a wider circumference, and as a result also have a greater internal area and a larger cuticle surface area. This generally makes them stronger and less susceptible to breakage.

FOLLICLE SIZE DETERMINES **HAIR THICKNESS**

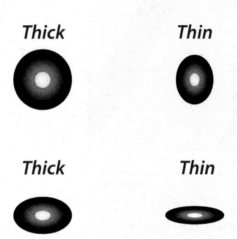

Knowing if your daughter has thin or thick strands will put you in good stead, especially if your goal is to grow her hair as long as possible. Generally speaking, thinner hair is weaker and takes more effort to stop from breaking, and thus it is harder for it to retain its length.

There is also a common saying in the natural community that "fine hair loves protein," and it may well be the case, because fine hair has less keratin than thicker hair and additional protein may be beneficial for strengthening it. We will learn how to check strand thickness and select appropriate products in more detail in the 'Choosing products' chapter.

CHAPTER 5 YOUR BABY'S HAIR 0 – 1 YEARS

WHAT TO EXPECT

The first year of a baby's life is an exciting time, and their hair will go through lots of changes. This period provides a great opportunity to start a strong foundation with a healthy hair care routine. My ethos is: It's never too early to start taking care of your daughter's hair. In fact, I started a healthy hair care routine with my daughter from day one.

During the first year of life as she develops, her hair is also developing. It will grow longer, get fuller in density and change in texture as time passes and she matures. None of this needs to be daunting; we just need to understand what to do at each stage.

AT BIRTH

In the womb, your daughter develops her hair follicles, and by the time she is born, they will already be in place. By approximately week 22, a foetus will have around five million hair follicles on its body, with a set amount on its head as determined by race. Studies have found that afro-textured hair has the lowest density, with approximately 190 hairs per square centimetre, compared to Caucasian hair, which has approximately 227 hairs in the same space.

Only the follicles are in place, not necessarily the hair strands. Genetics and health determine when the hair strands begin to grow from the follicles.

HAIR AT BIRTH

The number of actual hair strands (not follicles) that a baby is born with is again genetically determined. Some babies hit the hair lottery and are born with a full head of hair, while others have hardly any hair. It is impossible to predict with any accuracy how much will be present or what colour or texture the hair will be at birth.

Regardless of how much hair your daughter is born with, it's important to start a hair care routine as soon as possible in order to (A) get into the habit and to (B) create the optimum environment for her hair to thrive, because you simply don't know how close the hair beneath the skin is to growing out.

SKULL AT BIRTH

Babies are born with two soft spots on their heads, called fontanelles. The back soft spot, triangular in shape, is called the posterior fontanelle and is normally the smaller of the two. The soft spot at the front is called the anterior fontanelle, and is larger and diamond in shape.

Babies are born with these so that their head shape can mould as they are passing through the birth canal. It is nature's way of making their heads temporarily smaller.

These fontanelles fuse and close over time. The back fontanelle will normally close when the child is 6-8 weeks old, and the front fontanelle will normally close fully at around 18 months. Hence, in the first years of life we must be extremely delicate when caring for our daughters' hair as their skulls are fragile and need a very soft touch!

HAIR DENSITY AT BIRTH

From my own personal observations, babies at birth generally tend to fall into the following categories.

FULL HAIR

A baby born with a full head of hair will have hair that covers the majority of their scalp.

FINE HAIR

Babies can also be born with very fine hair, so fine that it may appear to be bald, but upon closer inspection, short, fine hairs will be visible.

BALD HAIR

Babies can also be born with little to no visible hair on their head. It is important to remember that if this is the case, the infant will have all their hair follicles in place under the skin.

PATCHY HAIR

Some babies are born without uniformity in the hair length. So it can seem longer in places and appear bald in others.

No matter how much hair they have at birth, the density of their hair will likely increase as their follicles mature and grow hair. Hair strands that were fine at birth will grow thicker over time.

The hair growth rate is determined by hormones, and it's important to note that some babies will in fact lose all of their hair in the first six months of life due to them entering the telegen/shed phase in their hair cycle.

If this happens to your baby, don't freak out. It's normal. The good news is that babies will likely enter the anagen/growth phase very quickly afterwards.

HAIR TEXTURE AT BIRTH

When babies are born, their hair will generally be at its finest and softest. Many babies who will later develop afro-textured hair will be born with wavy, curly and sometimes straight hair.

It's important to be aware and understand in advance that your baby's hair texture will change, and as it does so will the needs of her hair.

It's also equally important to not get too attached to one type of hair texture. It's really sad, but in my personal observation with having a girl, there can be extreme scrutiny in the black community on hair texture and hair texture changes.

Some people even see hair texture change as a negative thing.

When my daughter was around 6 months old, she had around 3-4" of soft curly hair, which I would often style in sleek bunches as that was a quick, easy and cute style. With this style, we went to a baby shower and met a woman who commented on how "pretty and soft and **good**" her hair was. I felt uncomfortable with her mentality and proceeded to explain that I had used a hair-curling product to emphasize and define the curls in her hair, making small talk.

Then, around a year later, we went to another function. I had again styled my daughter's hair into bunches, but this time they were not sleek because her hair texture had changed to be more afro in texture and it wasn't a suited to sleek styles.

Low and behold, enter the same woman. The first thing she said to me, before even saying "hello" or "how are you," was "Her hair's changed. When did that happen?" With a look of disappointment on her face, I could again tell by her tone that she was implying Bae's hair had somehow turned 'bad' because it was was now more afro in texture.

I didn't bother responding.

Did she really expect me to come up with the exact date that Bae's hair had changed? I think I said something along the lines of "Yeah, it's changed now, it looks so cute today!" to let her know that I wasn't ashamed or unhappy with how her hair was progressing.

It was such an ignorant question, but it highlighted the all too common attitudes towards hair types. While outlooks on natural hair in the black community are changing for the better, it is important to be aware of the shortcomings we still face in our community.

TEXTURE ESTABLISHMENT

I call the transition to more afro-textured hair 'texture establishment.' The changes in hair texture is just the journey hair will take towards its end texture.

It's quite a journey that black hair texture can take, and for my daughter we went through around 4-5 textures before we arrived at her established texture. We went from straight to wavy to curly to more curly to afro.

At each stage, her hair had different requirements, but my general thinking is that as the hair texture gets curlier, it also gets drier and needs more moisture.

It's important to note here that hair texture changes are caused by hormones and are totally normal. Generally, afro hair follows the trajectory of straighter to curlier, but a whole host of things can happen when a mix of environment, diet and genetics surround a child's development. Some babies' hair can change texture from curly to straight. An infant's hair colour can even change throughout infantile development, going from light to dark or dark to light. Scientists don't fully know the causation, but the fact is, this is all normal!

The key to navigating this journey successfully is in being receptive to the changes and being flexible. The hair will have different needs as it changes, so we must stay open-minded and ready to adapt our hair care practices as required.

LET IT GO

First and foremost, we need to get comfortable with the idea of change. We need to accept that hair texture will likely change, just like everything else in life.

We should never stay mentally fixated on a particular texture and merely hope that the hair stays like that. There is no product, no oil, no conditioner that can keep your child's hair at a particular stage of its development. So let that one go, and let the hair do its thing. It has a life of its own and needs to live. Your part is in facilitating its life.

Because your daughter's hair will change the most in its first year, I have broken down its stages to give you some guidance in expectations:

MONTHS 1-3

The hair will likely be at its softest at this time. It will tend to have a lot of natural sheen and can feel hydrated without the use of additional moisturizers.

The curl pattern will generally be much looser and straighter, and you will notice with time how the hair will get wavier and curlier, potentially losing some natural sheen.

During these three months of life, you generally do not need to do much with the hair besides maintaining its hydration. I recommend using water followed by olive oil. You will need to keep the hair hydrated, regardless of how moisturized it appears.

TOP TIP

Appearance only tells half of the story. During this period, the hair may be very shiny and look very moisturized, but this may be due to its exposure to amniotic fluid for a prolonged period of time. This fluid offers continuous hydration when present, but after birth it will eventually dry out. Hence, your goal is to substitute and maintain moisture levels.

CRADLE CAP

Seborrheic dermatitis or cradle cap is a common condition that usually appears in babies aged 1–3 months. It is generally harmless and can appear as large, greasy, yellow or brown scales on your baby's scalp. Its exact cause is not completely clear, yet some theorize that it stems from a temporary hormone imbalance that can cause the sebaceous glands to go into overdrive, producing excess sebum, which then dries and crusts.

It is not contagious, but it can be distressing for mothers. You generally don't need to see your doctor unless it becomes inflamed or spreads to other body parts.

TREATING CRADLE CAP

The temptation to flake it off the scalp is real. I know, because when my daughter had cradle cap, I had to fight the urge of doing it myself. There is a better way, which I used to eliminate my daughter's cradle cap quickly and efficiently.

Step 1

Warm 2-3 tablespoons of extra virgin olive oil in a pan over a low heat. Do not let it get hot; only warm it to a temperature that your baby can tolerate easily. You can test the temperature by putting some on the back of your hand.

Step 2

Transfer the oil to a bowl and, using a cotton wool ball, gently dab it onto the affected area.

Step 3

Gently rub it in in circular motions with a soft baby brush, the cotton wool or the pads of your fingers.

Step 4

No flaking or scratching. Use a tissue to dab the excess oil from the hair if necessary.

Step 5

Repeat this daily. You will find that over time, the scales will loosen and come away by the time you reach Step 3. Repeat this until the patch is gone.

It worked brilliantly for us and got rid of the cradle cap in less than a week!

MONTHS 3–6

At this point, the hair is likely to begin or advance in its journey towards its curlier texture. During this period, it is likely that you will need to modify your approach towards the hair as its needs change. Now is a good time to introduce a conditioner and leave-in conditioner into your hair care routine.

The curlier the hair, the drier it can be. I recommend upgrading from using just water to moisturize the hair to using water mixed with either a leave-in conditioner for infants or aloe vera juice.

Following either application, olive oil should also be applied. Shampoo is optional, but if you do decide to use it, then apply olive oil to the hair beforehand to prevent the shampoo from stripping or dying the hair.

DRY PATCHES

During this tender age, you need to be alert and identify any dry patches of hair immediately. The majority of my daughter's hair maintained moisture, but there was a patch of hair in her crown that seemed to dry out immediately after moisturizing and sealing. This patch of hair had much less sheen than the rest and it tangled constantly. My fear with the dry patch was that it was going to break off, leaving her with a bald or shorter patch on the crown. If you encounter the same, please see the solution in the 'Common issues and FAQs' chapter.

MONTHS 6–12

This period of my daughter's hair journey was where challenges became apparent. The styles I was using prior to this stopped working altogether.

I generally wore her hair all out with a cute bow on the side. I did not braid it, but instead would wet it, put in leave-in conditioner and use a soft brush to style it, finishing off with the bow. It was pretty simple. At six months, her afro seemingly popped out overnight, and this style was no longer an option as her hair was now prone to tangling and dryness.

If this is also the case for you, then I recommend starting to cornrow or plait the hair. It doesn't have to be anything elaborate. Just an easy-to-do, loose and cute style. Don't worry if you don't know how; you will learn what to do in the 'Braiding and cornrowing' chapter.

PRODUCTS LAYERING

The hair is generally getting curlier at this stage, and I definitely noticed that it was much more prone to dryness than previously. If you are noticing drier hair, then I recommend introducing product layering into your hair care routine. Please see the 'Product layering' chapter for a full explanation.

DRYING

It can be tempting at this time to start using a blow-dryer on your daughter's hair, as it will likely be longer and thicker at this time, but my advice is to avoid the hairdryer as it can cause dryness and damage.

What you can try instead is gently towel-drying the hair and then braiding it while still damp or banding it, which will be explained later.

TOP TIP

My main piece of advice for you during your daughter's first year is to enjoy this tender time, including the changes in her hair. Always remember your number one priority is to keep it moisturized.

As we progress onto years one to two, moisturizing will remain a priority. It is the KEY to healthy and long hair, so better to start sooner rather than later!

CHAPTER 6   YOUR BABY'S HAIR 1 – 2 YEARS

HAIR AT ONE: **WHAT TO EXPECT?**

When dealing with kinky, curly and afro hair, you will find that hair care in years 1 to 2 is a completely different ball game than previously. The hair will be longer, thicker, curlier and more prone to tangling and dryness than before.

What this means for mothers is that it will take more time and energy to do.

Before they turn one, baby's hairstyles are generally quite quick and easy to put together. You might leave the hair free, put a cute hairband or bow into the hair or maybe put it into bunches. But after hitting the one-year mark, the hair begins to make its own new, fussy demands.

TEXTURE CHANGES

Besides your child talking more, walking and developing a personality, the hair also begins to exhibit some changes. In a way, you could say its personality also starts to take flight. The texture will have changed significantly from when she was first born. This will vary depending on what her ultimate texture will be, but any curls will likely have tightened to some degree.

Just as your daughter begins to enjoy some food over others, favours particular food types or claps to a particular song, the hair also gets pickier—and rightfully so! This is a time when you will also need to make a shift and pay attention to what your daughter's hair likes and dislikes.

HAIR DRYNESS

Hair may transition into a drier state, and maintaining its moisture may prove difficult.

At this stage, you will need to pull together your staple product arsenal and begin to incorporate more products into your regime. You may have to look into a deep conditioner, a leave-in conditioner and a daily moisturizer to keep hair health optimized.

PRODUCT SELECTION

You will need to be very receptive, product-wise, going forwards. Be open to the fact that what once worked may not work now.

You now need to look for products that offer your daughter's hair the following:

1 – Moisture

2 – Adequate sealing in of moisture

3 – Slip for aid with detangling

We talk more about product selection in detail later, especially in regards to what substances work best with certain types of hair. You will now start to identify products that work particularly well with your daughter's hair, and do not be scared of experimenting.

THERE WILL BE NEW AREAS OF HAIR GROWTH

Do you recall that a baby is born with all of his or her hair follicles? Well, now is the time she will start to sprout new hair in new places!

You will notice new hair in the hairline, especially in the temples and at the nape. Even if this hair is fresh, it should not be ignored with the hope that it grows quickly to meet the rest of the hair. We have all seen babies with their hair in bunches, with very short hair in the hairline that doesn't reach all the way to the bunch. The short hair may stick up and may even be texturally different to the rest of the hair in the bunch. It is possible that this hair isn't broken, but is in fact new hair growing in.

I can remember putting my daughter's hair in bunches and realizing the hair at the nape did not reach as it had previously. I got really worried that I had damaged her hair, but upon closer inspection, I realized that it was in fact new growth. This is something that deserves your special attention and notice.

This new growth is delicate and needs a soft touch. It needs to catch up to the rest of the hair; hence, we need to effectively identify it and make sure it doesn't get neglected and is conditioned and moisturized with the rest of the hair.

PROTECTIVE STYLES WILL BE YOUR KEY

Protective hairstyles are going to be your key in years one to two. You will read about them later in this book, but as a general rule, they are styles that protect the hair from breakage so it can retain length.

I started to cornrow my daughter's hair on and off from when she was 9 months old. But in years one to two, I did it consistently for the entire year! I just wanted to protect her hair and focus on it growing. She only wore it out on special occasions, and I can report this is the year she made the most length gains thus far.

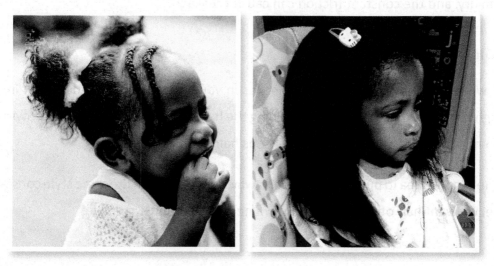

1st birthday left picture, 2nd birthday right picture.

CHOOSING A PROTECTIVE STYLE

I would advise you to transition into implementing a protective hairstyle for your daughter's hair to achieve maximum growth in years 1-2.

It can sometimes be a mental adjustment, especially if you are used to your daughter's hair being out. You need to also take into account the extra time needed to maintain a protective style.

The following styles are great for this age group, since they reduce stress on the hair and keep hair off the body and clothing.

CORNROWS

Cornrows are a good option for protective styling. However, please keep in mind that hair should not be cornrowed down towards the shoulders, where it will rub on her neck or clothes.

Instead, cornrow the hair going up into bunches or a ponytail, because when the hair touches clothing, the clothes can absorb moisture from the ends of the hair, making them dry, and the constant friction can cause breakage.

AVOID REPETITIVE STYLING

You will need to have 2–3 protective styles in your arsenal to keep good faith in your daughter's hair. You want to avoid stressing the hair through repetitive styling. Switching it up not only gives variety, but also it keeps hair healthy!

It's not a good idea to pull the hair up and away from the face in the same style constantly. Sure, we want hair off of clothing, but we need to get a little creative.

From my own experience, using the same style repetitively can lead to damage. I got a bit stuck in a style rut with my daughter's hair and would constantly cornrow her hair into bunches. The stress of this created a small, thin patch of hair at the back. Always remember that young hair is delicate!

You need to be vigilant when styling your daughter's hair and check for any damaged, bald or thin spots. If you do notice any, then you need to evaluate whether the style is causing damage and either modify that particular style or switch to another.

DON'T PLAIT TOO SMALL OR TOO TIGHT

Avoid super small plaits because they can be a nightmare to take out of a fidgety baby's hair. We want to keep the manipulation of the hair as low as we can, so always aim to do plaits that you can remove pretty easily.

Similarly, don't plait too tight, because this will cause bald spots, and many can speak to this. You want to aim to do loose, large plaits.

WHAT IF MY DAUGHTER DOESN'T WEAR PLAITS?

It may be that your daughter doesn't wear plaits or twists at this time, which is absolutely fine. If this is the case, try to keep the hair off the clothes whenever possible by creating loose bunches, buns or ponytails. Always keep the ends of the hair moisturized!

WASHING THE HAIR WILL TAKE LONGER

Another change you will encounter is the time needed to wash your daughter's hair. It will no longer be an afterthought and will require active planning.

THE FIGHT

Okay, so let me be real. Washing hair can be a battle, and I discovered this with my daughter when she finally had the strength to resist the routine.

When she was a baby and couldn't wriggle that much and wasn't strong, it was easy to get away with washing her hair without much fuss. But when she turned one and was growing increasingly curious, the entire process became an ordeal. I'd wash her hair and she would wriggle and squirm, try to grab my hair, her hair; she even tried to eat the shampoo! I was holding her and washing her hair in the sink at this time, using a jug to pour water over her hair, which was tricky. I was juggling my slippery child while trying to wash her, and all the while she was busy wiggling about.

If you are also washing your child's hair in the sink, I'd advise you to use the technique specified in the 'washing' chapter later in this book to make your life much easier!

YOU MAY HAVE TO CHANGE THE WAY YOU DRY THE HAIR

Another consideration that you'll have to make will be to think more about how you will dry your daughter's hair. I've said it before and I'll say it again: don't use a blow dryer on your daughter's hair consistently, because it will eventually lead to breakage.

Instead, a great alternative is banding, which helps the hair dry stretched for easy styling. You can read how to band in the 'Techniques' chapter. You should try it for heatless stretching.

DO HER HAIR IN HER HIGH CHAIR

If you have been doing your daughter's hair on your lap, now is the time to switch to a high chair. One-year-olds are notoriously difficult to keep still, and it can be exhausting. High chairs are the solution.

They can colour in, read a book or watch a video while restrained, which should keep them entertained and safe while you get to work.

HAIR TIME IS HAPPY TIME

However you do your daughter's hair, you need to make sure that hair time is a happy and not a stressful time. Make it fun, light and enjoyable for everyone.

If she's really not into something, don't force it. Take breaks where necessary, laugh, cuddle and kiss her where you can. The ultimate goal of this approach, after all, is for your daughter to have a positive connection with hair time.

CHAPTER 7 TODDLERS AND YOUNG CHILDREN

HAIR AT TWO AND BEYOND: **WHAT TO EXPECT**

If you found caring for your daughter's hair challenging in years 1–2, you may find that caring for a toddler's hair is much easier. I know I did. By this time you will be situated with the texture and characteristics of her hair, and going forwards you begin to feel confident.

HER TEXTURE SHOULD BE ESTABLISHED

You will find it easier because her hair texture is now less likely to change and should be nearly established with a final texture. This is good news. It means you no longer have to manage major texture changes. Instead, you get to focus on learning what products and ingredients work for her hair in the long term.

Another benefit of her hair texture stabilizing is that you will now know what hair type she is. This knowledge alone can help hair care management and planning.

IDENTIFY YOUR DAUGHTER'S HAIR TYPE

When her hair texture has stopped changing, it's a good time to evaluate her hair to get an idea of her hair type.

The best way to do this is on dry, 'naked' hair: that is, hair that has no product in it. I would advise you to wash and condition the hair as usual, but rinse the conditioner out fully and let the hair dry naturally without product. Some products can cause the curls in the hair to 'pop' or stand out more, but we need to see what the hair does on its own.

You can then compare her texture to the hair type pictures in the 'hair science' chapter to discover which she is.

You will likely discover that she has two or even three textures, which is completely normal. Most of us actually have two textures of hair. My daughter has two distinct textures. Her hair has looser curls around the perimeter, but at the crown, the curls are a lot tighter.

Hair typing isn't an exact science, so you may be slightly off, but it will give you an idea and this can help you understand her hair more.

MANAGING TWO HAIR TYPES

If you discover that your daughter does indeed have 2 hair textures, then you are not alone, and it's actually easy to manage, although it can seem daunting if they are very different.

The key thing to remember in this scenario is that the curlier the hair, the more delicate and prone to dryness it will be. Focus on keeping the driest parts of the hair hydrated; this should ensure that you keep ALL of the hair hydrated.

STYLING HAIR WITH TWO TEXTURES

There are some considerations that will need to be made when styling hair with two textures. I have found it good practice to use additional product layers on drier sections of hair to really lock the moisture in place where it is needed.

For example, if you are dealing with a dry patch, then I would suggest using a heavier oil or cream on that patch, but you can read the complete solution in the 'Common issues and FAQs' chapter.

It can be easy to dismiss a dry patch as just that. But dismissing it can only worsen the inconsistencies in hair moisture across the different textures of your child's hair. You should aim to hydrate the dry patch and eradicate it. Accepting a dry patch is dangerous because it shows complacency, which is never good in a healthy hair care regime.

TOP TIP

As a general rule when selecting products, you want to choose products that leave the hair feeling moisturized and with a natural sheen when dry.

FIND WHAT YOUR DAUGHTER'S HAIR LOVES

Now that you are searching for staple products, I have some advice for you. Don't just go for products that her hair likes; search instead for products that her hair absolutely loves! Find products that will bring out the absolute best in her hair. To identify these, I advise you to create a hair journal. This will help you because you are likely to experiment with lots of products and you want to keep track so you don't forget anything and can easily go back and find the good ones.

AN EXAMPLE OF A HAIR JOURNAL

A hair journal is not a complicated document at all; simply put, it's a diary where you make notes on hair products you have tried and their results.

So you will want to make notes on the following:

The product

Its key ingredients

Does it offer slip?

Does the hair feel moisturized after use?

Does the hair have natural sheen after use?

An example journal:

PRODUCT	KEY INGREDIENTS	SLIPPERY	MOISTURE?	SHEEN?
Conditioner A	Aloe vera, honey	No	Yes	No
Conditioner B	Jojoba oil, coconut oil	Yes	Yes	Yes

The above is just an example, but hopefully you get the idea. This will become a go-to resource for you when evaluating products and whether to reuse them. Also, by noting the key ingredients, you will be able to identify the actual ingredients that work well for your daughter, which is good knowledge to have on your continued journey.

WHY SLIP, MOISTURE AND SHEEN?

The key metrics I advise you to measure when assessing products are the 'slip, moisture and sheen,' or SMS, they offer the hair. This is because these three elements are beneficial to healthy hair.

Slip – The more slippery a product makes the hair feel, the easier the hair will be to detangle which will result in less breakage.

Moisture – Our aim is to keep the hair as hydrated as possible to stop the breakage the can stem from dryness.

Sheen – We want the hair to have a natural sheen and not look visibly dry.

You need to make sure you are constantly monitoring the hair, because we want to make sure we continue to make health and length gains and not suffer any setbacks.

TOP TIP

Any product you are using that leads the hair to feel dry after use is likely not a good product. With a conditioner, for example, if after it is washed out the hair feels rough or dry, it's likely not a good one, because a good conditioner will leave the hair feeling soft and hydrated.

MONITOR THE OVERALL HEALTH OF THE HAIR

Along with monitoring the products you use, it is also good practice to monitor the overall health of the hair and discover if there are any damaged or vulnerable areas. You need to check the ends of the hair for damage or splits.

Hair damage is likely to occur at the ends of the hair, as these are the oldest, driest and most vulnerable parts; if damage is found, then it not only needs to be removed, but its cause should be identified and eradicated. There is absolutely no point in ignoring damaged areas, because they won't just go away and will only get worse.

SETBACKS

A setback is an event in your daughter's hair journey that takes her back a step or two. The most common setback being damaged ends that need to be cut off.

If you think about it, hair will grow on average 6" a year, so if your daughter has a setback that causes 3" to be cut off, then we are set back and lose 6 months of progress, which in my eyes is a lot.

I'm not saying you should hang on to the damaged ends in order to keep the length, as I believe healthy hair is the number one priority, but I am saying that you should try to avoid setbacks by following healthy hair care practices in the first instance.

CUTTING THE HAIR

To cut or not to cut? That is the question.

I'm often asked about cutting and trimming the hair, and there are lots of different schools of thought on this. My advice is this: *trim the hair only when necessary.*

As we know, hair beyond the follicle is dead.

The common myth that cutting the hair makes it grow faster is not true. It's not possible for hair that has been cut to communicate in any way to its follicles and ask them to grow hair faster, so the rate of hair growth will remain the same. It's just not essential to cut the hair if it's not damaged.

SEARCH AND DESTROY

Instead of cutting the hair, a great way to maintain healthy ends is to use the search and destroy method. This is the practice of cutting only damaged hair, leaving healthy hair intact.

HOW TO SEARCH AND DESTROY

It's a great method because it allows you to maintain healthy ends while minimizing sacrifices in overall length.

The best way I have found to do this method is by working in small sections and doing the following on dry, stretched hair:

1) Part the hair into four sections down the middle and from ear to ear, clipping three sections away.

2) Using a rat-tail comb on the loose section, part horizontally so you are working with a section about 1" deep; clip the rest away.

3) Hold a white sheet of paper behind the ends of the hair to help you see better and inspect the hair for the following:

    - Split ends

    - Single strand knots

    - Broken ends

4) If you find any, cut them out!

To do this, I recommend you invest in some hair cutting scissors, as they are sharp and leave the ends with a nice, clean finish. Blunt scissors can leave the ends of the hair slightly frayed. Think of sharp versus blunt scissors on fabric to get more of an idea.

I would also recommend you to do this every six months.

If your daughter has more severe damage and her hair has to be cut, I recommend you visit a reputable stylist to get the job done. I would not recommend you do this yourself!

What you might want to do prior to the appointment is wash, condition and stretch your daughters' hair, because we know some stylists can be heavy-handed, which is not good. But leave the cutting to the professional.

When explaining to your stylist, specify why you are cutting the hair, and the MAXIMUM amount that should be cut off. Be very specific to not only establish expectations, but also accountability with the stylist. Stylists often like to take matters into their own hands and get scissor-happy. You have to be firm and clearly state what you want.

You, more than anyone, know exactly how much hair damage your daughter has. You know exactly what needs to come off.

HAIR GOALS

As I mentioned in an earlier chapter, having a healthy hair goal is very important. But for some of us, a health goal is compounded by a length goal we want our daughters to achieve. It specifies how long we want our daughters' hair to be and in what timeframe. As we progress onto having young children, we can really start to systematically move towards these goals.

When setting a hair length goal, it's important to have a justification. Why do you want long and healthy hair for your daughter? It's very personal, so it doesn't have to be something you share with everyone. The important thing is to remain motivated if you experience any setbacks.

LENGTH CHECK

A good way to check where you are in relation to your goals is through doing a length check. This generally involves straightening the hair to some degree so you can see its stretched length.

Since I don't advocate blow-drying or straightening the hair often, a length check should be done once or twice a year. I find it preferable to do this check on a special occasion as that is when I'm more likely to straighten my daughter's hair.

With the shrinkage associated with afro hair, progress is not easily identified. Yes, you can get random bits of hair and stretch these out to get a general idea of the length, but it doesn't give the complete picture.

HOW TO DO A LENGTH CHECK

Heat application to a child's hair can cause damage, but if we take precautions, we can minimize that risk.

Here's how I recommend doing a length check:

1) Wash and deep condition the hair as normal, but rinse out all of the conditioner completely.

2) Apply a leave-in conditioner, followed by a heat protectant. Band the hair in 8–12 sections, and let it dry completely, preferably overnight.

3) Remove the bands, and in small sections, flat iron the hair on a low setting, being sure to only do 2 passes per section of hair. Use the comb and chase method to get the hair as straight as possible.

4) Repeat until all of the hair is straightened, and then you will see the stretched length.

5) Take a picture!

Pictures are a fantastic way to see progress over time. It can often be that we feel we are making no progress, but pictures will tell the full story!

MEASURING

I'd also advise measuring the hair at least once a year so you become familiar with your daughter's growth rate; the length check is the ideal time to do this also.

It's really simple to do. I advise using a cloth tape measure, placing it at the base of the hair on the scalp and measuring down the length of the strand. This should be done annually so you have a record of your daughter's progress.

CARING FOR THE HAIR AT NIGHT

It's important to also now think about building a full regime, and that includes considerations for how to protect the hair at night while your daughter is asleep.

A satin pillowcase is a great tool in any hair care regime, because it limits the amount of moisture lost through absorption into cotton sheets.

It's not essential for everyone, but for children with chronically dry hair, I suggest it. I use it for my daughter and I have seen a marked improvement in her hair's moisture levels. It's definitely something to consider, and combined with protective styles, it offers maximum protection to the hair strands.

PROTECTIVE STYLES FOR TODDLERS AND YOUNG CHILDREN

You may be wondering what protective styles I recommend, so I've dedicated a few chapters to them. You can read more in the 'Protective styling' and the 'Braiding and twisting' chapters. I've got you covered!

ENJOY HER HAIR!!!

It is important to reiterate that you should have fun with your daughter's hair going forward in its growth.

Yes, you may hit bumps in the road and the odd setback, but the important thing to remember is that she is young and impressionable. She will pick up on any negative vibes you are giving out. If you are approaching her hair as a chore, then she too will begin to treat it as such. Enjoy hair time and make it a reflection of her personality and interests. Not only will she begin to take control of her own self-image, but she will associate your presence and participation as support of who she is.

CHAPTER 8 PRODUCTS

HAIR CARE PRODUCT SELECTION

Now's the time we can delve deeper into the often confusing and sometimes misleading world of hair products.

The truth is, correct product selection is a foundational element to any healthy hair care regime. It is so vitally important that I would venture to say that without the correct products, it would be extremely difficult for your daughter to have healthy hair. That is because the correct products will give the hair what it needs to stay moisturized, strong and damage-free.

I would highly recommend selecting products for a child's hair that are organic or natural. Harsh chemicals are often bad for the hair and can cause irritation. It is best to avoid these types.

It's important to begin to understand product ingredients and formations so you can know what to buy and why. The claims a product makes in its marketing can become easily distracting, and preparation and knowledge when entering the marketplace for hair care products is crucial.

ALWAYS THINK MOISTURE

Moisturizing afro hair is a priority for this hair type. Hair products are notorious for sinfully robbing the hair and even preventing hydration. Hence, I will help you actively seek out products that will increase moisture levels. Protein is also important to hair health, but that will be discussed in detail in the next chapter.

WHY CORRECT PRODUCT SELECTION IS IMPORTANT

It's important to understand ingredients because hair products are something we cannot live without, and we need to know if what we are using is beneficial or detrimental to hair.

We need to remember that **hair damage happens slowly,** and if we use products that do not give the hair the moisture and strength it needs, over time brittle, breaking hair will result.

WHAT IS A STAPLE PRODUCT?

Staple products are essential products in your hair care arsenal that must be consistently used to keep hair clean, conditioned and moisturized.

STAPLE PRODUCTS FOR HEALTHY HAIR

> Shampoo

> Conditioner

> Leave-in conditioner

> Oil

> Moisturizer

> Hair butter (or heavy cream)

Understanding the significance of these resources will validate the reasoning behind their importance.

PRODUCTS EXPLAINED

SHAMPOO

Purpose

Shampoo is primarily used to clean the hair and scalp, removing dirt and product build-up. Secondary functions of shampoo also include improving the condition and appearance of the hair while also enhancing manageability.

The multitude of shampoos can be daunting. An entire aisle is dedicated to shampoo alone. While some add volume, others are for colour-treated hair. Some address split ends, while others claim to restore the hair. For our purposes, we only need to concern ourselves with two types: normal and clarifying shampoos.

Normal shampoo is used most commonly to generally clean and lightly condition the hair. Clarifying shampoo can be used to remove product build-up such as gel, silicones and waxes. However, with children's hair, it should not be necessary to use a clarifying shampoo often unless you frequently use gels, pomades or products with silicone.

A child does not have to cleanse the hair with shampoo frequently at all. Many shampoos (even the mild ones) are just too harsh for delicate afro hair, so an alternative is to wash the hair with a conditioner.

Co-washing

Conditioner washing or co-washing is popular because conditioners do not contain the harsh detergents of shampoos and therefore do not strip the hair of its natural oils. They do have some cleansing capabilities, and this is what makes co-washing safe, even over longer periods of time.

It is especially suitable for children because of its moisture retention properties. If your daughter has extremely dry hair, co-washing with a natural conditioner might be a good option.

Shampoo key ingredients:

Cleansing agents

Also known as surfactants or detergents; sulphates are traditionally the key surfactants in commercial shampoos. Yet we should pursue other natural options where possible.

Examples:

Chemical surfactants, anything ending in sulphate, e.g., Sodium lauryl sulphate (SLS), ammonium laureth sulphate.

More natural surfactants: Coco betaine, cocoamphoacetate.

Skin conditioners/Emollients/Oils/Lipids

These ingredients will sooth the scalp and skin and form a protective layer on hair strands, increasing manageability.

Examples:

Chemical ingredients: Mineral oil, paraffin oil, lanolin, chetyl alcohol, stearyl alcohol, dimethicone, amodimethicone, cyclomethicone.

Natural ingredients: Argan oil, coconut oil, avocado oil.

Moisturisers

Humectants are used as moisturizers in shampoo. They work by pulling water molecules from the environment into the hair shaft.

Examples: Anything that contains 'glycol' in the name e.g. propylene glycol and panthenol, sorbitol, sodium lactate.

Natural ingredients: aloe vera, vegetable glycerin/glycerol.

Preservatives

Preservatives increase the shelf life of a product.

Examples: Any type of paraben, e.g., methylparaben, propylparaben.

Natural preservatives: Sodium benzoate, benzoic acid.

Emulsifiers/Thickeners

The primary function of an emulsifier is to create a stable product blend whereby ingredients that do not mix naturally are able to combine, such as oil and water.

Examples: Lecithin, polysorbate, chetyl alcohol.

Natural Ingredient: Castor oil

CONDITIONER

Purpose

The function of a conditioner is to minimize hair damage and breakage by strengthening and moisturizing hair. A conditioner will aim to make the hair shinier, softer, smoother to touch and easier to comb.

There are typically three types of conditioner you will come across. Each will have a place in your daughter's hair care regime. These are instant, deep and leave-in conditioners.

Instant conditioner

These have no penetrating abilities and are generally left on the hair for a few minutes. They are applied to smooth and coat the hair. Instant conditioners are ideal to use when detangling hair because they make the hair very slippery and easy to work with. It is not possible to deep condition hair with an instant conditioner, even if you leave it on for an extended period of time.

Deep conditioner

A deep conditioner is one that is designed to penetrate into the hair shaft and have more lasting results. They will typically be moisture- or protein-focused and will either hydrate or strengthen the hair. They are usually left on the hair for an extended period of time, 20–30 minutes, and can be used with heat for maximum penetration.

Leave-in conditioner

Leave-in conditioners are not rinsed out of the hair and their primary function is to moisturize the hair, add slip to aid with detangling and maximize the benefits of prior conditioning. They will contain a mix of moisturizing and strengthening ingredients and will help hair hold in moisture.

Conditioners key ingredients:

Moisturizers

Humectants are used as moisturizers in conditioner. They work by pulling water molecules from the environment into the hair shaft.

Examples: Anything that contains 'glycol' in the name e.g. propylene glycol and panthenol, sorbitol, sodium lactate.

Natural ingredients: Aloe vera, vegetable glycerine/glycerol.

Reconstructors

Protein conditioners will normally contain a hydrolysed protein to penetrate the hair shaft and add strength from within.

Examples: Anything starting with hydrolysed, e.g., hydrolysed keratin, hydrolysed silk protein and amino acids.

Acidifiers

These are used to adjust the PH level in conditioner to make it more acid or alkali.

Examples: Citric acid, ascorbic acid, sodium hydroxide.

Skin conditioners/Emollients/Oils/Lipids

These ingredients will sooth the scalp and skin and form a protective layer on hair strands increasing manageability.

Examples:

Chemical ingredients: Mineral oil, paraffin oil, lanolin, chetyl alcohol, stearyl alcohol, dimethicone, amodimethicone, cyclomethicone.

Natural ingredients: Argan oil, coconut oil, avocado oil.

Thermal protectors

Silicones are used in conditioners for their smoothing and also heat protecting properties.

Examples: Anything ending in cone, e.g., dimethicone, amodimethicone, cyclomethicone.

Oils and butters

Natural oils and butters are used for their hair conditioning benefits.

Examples: Coconut oil, argan oil, extra virgin olive oil, shea butter, avocado butter.

Preservatives

Preservatives increase the shelf life of a product.

Examples: Any type of paraben, e.g., methyl paraben, propyl paraben.

Natural preservatives: Sodium benzoate, benzoic acid.

Emulsifiers/Thickeners

The primary function of an emulsifier is to create a stable product blend whereby ingredients that do not mix naturally are able to combine, such as oil and water.

Examples: Lecithin, polysorbate, chetyl alcohol.

Natural ingredient: Castor oil

OIL

Purpose

In a healthy hair care regime, oil is used primarily as a sealant or a conditioner. Oils are great for natural hair because most are rich in vitamins and essential fatty acids and they condition, smooth and soften hair and can help to prevent hair weakening from washing which is known as hydral fatigue.

Oils can be broken down into those that are able to penetrate the hair and those that are not.

Oils that penetrate the hair

Chemically speaking, oils can be broken down into two categories: saturated (straight chain) and unsaturated (multiple chains). Typically, the straight chains of saturated oils can be absorbed easier into the hair shaft. That's not to say that they can moisturize like water, but they can deliver their benefits directly to the hair cortex.

Saturated oil examples

Coconut oil

Palm oil

Non-saturated oil examples

Mineral oil

Castor oil

Olive oil

Saturated oils can be used in a healthy hair regime to combat hydral fatigue, which is the damage caused by the hair expanding and contracting to accommodate and release water when washing and drying.

WHAT IS HYDRAL FATIGUE?

A good way to think of it is like a damaged hairband. We stretch it to put it on, and then take it off and after repeated use the hairband will not shrink back to its original size.

It will have stretched and lost elasticity.

This is similar to the damage hydral fatigue can do; it can cause the hair to lose elasticity and not shrink back after being wet. This stretching affects the integrity of the hairs' cuticle and cortex, weakening them and resulting in porosity and breakage issues, which of course we need to avoid!

Saturated oils have been shown to have polar regions, which have an affinity towards the hairs' protein, keratin. So they are effective at combating hydral fatigue if they are applied before washing, as they will be absorbed into the hair shaft and will temporarily bond with the keratin in the hair. This will reduce the amount by which the hair swells thus reducing the risk of damage. It is a good idea to use an oil, such as coconut oil, as a pre-shampoo treatment to keep the hair as healthy as possible.

OILS FOR SEALING

Oils by nature repel water. Non-saturated and polar oils are great for sealing in moisture and not letting water out. Water-repelling oils can also be called occlusive or hydrophobic.

OIL AS A CONDITIONER

Oils are also used as conditioners; they can either be for pre-shampoo treatment to combat hydral fatigue as detailed above or for hot oil conditioning treatments to deliver other benefits such as strength, pliability, softness and shine.

OILS FOR SEALING AND THEIR PROPERTIES

Jojoba oil – contains meristic acid and vitamins A, B1, B6 and E. It closely resembles sebum, the hair's natural oil, and can add shine, elasticity and softness to the hair.

Grapeseed oil – contains linoleic acid, an omega-6 fatty acid that can help prevent against moisture loss.

Jamaican black castor oil – contains vitamin E and essential fatty acids, which can help to soften the hair. Its heavy consistency also works well for thick hair.

OILS FOR CONDITIONING AND THEIR PROPERTIES

Extra virgin olive oil – contains anti-oxidants to promote a healthy scalp and hair.

Coconut oil – contains lauric acid, a principle fatty acid that has an attraction to hair proteins and can strengthen hair.

Avocado oil – contains fatty acids and vitamins A, E and D, which strengthen and soften hair.

Oils for hair can be either natural or commercial. Commercial oils will also contain silicones, emulsifiers, fragrances and preservatives. Whenever possible, use natural, cold pressed, virgin oils.

Other oils that can be used in a healthy hair regime are essential oils. These earn their name because they contain the scent or essence of the plant they are extracted from. They are highly concentrated and have to be mixed with a non-essential oil before use on the hair or skin.

Some essential oils and their benefits:

Rosemary oil – can stimulate the scalp, address dandruff problems and combat a flaky scalp.

Peppermint oil – can help stimulate blood flow to the scalp, which helps the hair receive nourishment, resulting in hair growth.

Tea tree oil – is a great scalp treatment and can help keep the scalp free of bacterial and fungal problems.

MOISTURIZER

Purpose

In simple terms, moisturizing hair is the way we quench the hair's thirst. As a part of our everyday life, moisture naturally evaporates from hair strands. Moisturizing is the way we replace and replenish what has been lost.

Water is by far the best hair moisturizer because of its abilities to penetrate into the hair shaft and deliver its thirst-quenching benefits right to the core of hair. The only issue with water is that it evaporates rapidly. After it is gone, the hair will again be dry.

Ideally, the act of hair moisturizing needs to be twofold. Not only should it hydrate, but also it should also retain moisture in the hair without letting it evaporate too quickly.

Most moisturizing products in the market address this dual need. They contain water, humectants, and emollients for lightly sealing the moisture into the hair.

It is common for people to make their own moisturizing sprays; these will usually consist of water, humectants (e.g. aloe vera, glycerin) and possibly oils (rosemary, jojoba).

But they are also a popular commercial product and commercially will include extra ingredients, including additional moisturizers, emulsifiers, butters and, in some cases, reconstructors.

HAIR BUTTER

Purpose

Butters are used in healthy hair care regimes, primarily as a sealant to hold in moisture, as they provide a thick coating that does the job well.

Natural butters are great for hair and offer many health benefits, the key benefit coming from their inherent fatty acids. Fatty acids, simply put, are good fats. They are long chain lipid-carboxylic acids and benefit the hair by fighting off water loss while protecting and conditioning the hair. Some butters are also natural emollients and can help soothe and stimulate the scalp for healthy hair growth.

Butters consist of saturated fats and are able to penetrate hair strands more readily (than unsaturated fats) because they consist of straight chains that can be absorbed by hair fibres.

Typically they are used in 3 ways:

> Whipped butter

  This will normally be a blend of a few butters whipped together to form an easy to apply aerated, cream-like consistency.

> Solid butter

  Butters are solid at room temperature, so will normally have to be melted before use, and can be used as a conditioning treatment or as a sealant.

> Commercial

  Commercial butters will have natural ingredients combined with other oils, emollients, emulsifiers, fragrances and preservatives. They often have a cream-like consistency.

Some people with extremely dry hair find the inclusion of a hair butter into their regime to be the key to extremely moisturized hair. Butters are popular to use as the final product when using the LOC method, which we shall explain later in the book.

Some popular butters and their benefits:

Coconut oil – technically a butter as it's solid at room temperature, it's high in lauric acid, a principle fatty acid. It has an attraction to hair proteins and is able to penetrate the hair to bond with them, which in turn strengthens the hair.

Shea – contains stearic acid, which coats the hair shaft and conditions the hair.

Cocoa – contains linoleic acid, which is known for being a skin healer, hence soothing any scalp irritation.

Murumuru – contains meristic acid to offer lubrication, as it is easily absorbed into hair strands.

Mango – contains oleic acid, which helps keep hair moisturized by fighting off water loss.

It is very common for people to make their own whipped butters, and these will normally contain a selection of butters whipped with an essential oil, such as rosemary, as a preservative.

In the next chapter, we will learn how to pick the correct products to meet our own child's unique hair needs.

CHAPTER 9 CHOOSING THE BEST PRODUCTS FOR YOUR DAUGHTER

Our hair needs should be the only consideration when buying hair products; however, with all the advertisements and diverse claims, one can get tempted to buy just about anything.

Different ingredients deliver different benefits, and some ingredients can have a negative impact on the hair, so we need to choose wisely!

INGREDIENTS TO USE WITH CAUTION

Before we look at what ingredients we do want, it's important to understand the ingredients that need to be used with caution or even avoided.

SULFATES

Sodium Lauryl/Laureth Sulfate (SLS), Ammonium Lauryl sulfate (ALS)

Sulfates are detergents that are typically found in shampoos and any product that cleanses and produces suds. They should be avoided because they are extremely harsh, and they do more than just remove dirt and excess oil. They also strip the hair's natural oils, which makes the hair vulnerable to dryness.

PARABENS

Methylparaben, propylparabe, ethylparaben, butylparaben and isobutylparaben

Parabens are preservatives that inhibit the growth of bacteria, fungi and other microbes in hair products. They are the most widely used preservative in cosmetics and been used regularly for decades. Recently some hair experts have raised questions regarding the safety of synthetic parabens in potentially causing malignant breast tumours. They have pointed to the parabens in deodorants as migrating from the underarm to the breast. While causality was weak, it has caused enough alarm for people to seek more natural alternatives.

MINERAL OIL

Mineral oils are widely used in greases and pomades marketed towards 'ethnic hair.' They are not necessarily dangerous to healthy hair, but because of their long term presence on store shelves, people have become accustomed to using them without knowing how. Mineral oil is an occlusive agent, meaning that if applied to the hair directly, it will cause a near impenetrable moisture seal, not allowing moisture in or out. This is not necessarily negative, as usage can imply a positive benefit. But the real issue has been the way mineral oil is marketed to the ethnic hair care market, usually as 'moisturising.' Mineral oil does not moisturise, but instead creates a strong moisture seal. My advice is to avoid mineral oil in all products except a grease or heavy cream that you use for sealing only.

DIETHANOLAMINE (DEA)

These ingredients are primarily used as PH adjusters and lathering agents when combined with a detergent.

These ingredients can cause scalp irritation and allergic reactions, and they can also deplete keratin levels, which will result in dry, brittle and lifeless hair. A 1999 study by the National Toxicology Program in the US found a correlation between cancer and tumours in laboratory animals when they had the chemical directly applied. Although this has not been shown to affect humans, especially in the low doses typically found in our products, many natural products avoid it altogether.

PROPYLENE GLYCOL (PG)

Propylene glycol is an effective humectant that helps deliver moisture to the hair and skin. It serves a dual function as the product is an antifreeze, keeping products from freezing during shipping and storage. Within the natural community, the substance is debated in regards to the risks it may present. For some people it can it can irritate skin and cause allergic reactions, so if you use it, do take caution.

WAIT! BEFORE SELECTING PRODUCTS

Before any products are selected, it's important to know more about your daughter's hair. This is more relevant for toddlers and older children. For babies, it is best to keep it natural and focus on hydration.

In Chapter 6, we learned about hair science, including hair porosity and hair thickness. Now we will learn how to evaluate these to help us select the most suitable products for our daughters.

TESTING FOR HAIR POROSITY

Testing for porosity will let us know if our daughters' hair porosity is high, medium or low, and will reveal more about her hair care needs.

HOW TO CHECK IT

The easiest way to test for hair porosity is by doing the float test, which is pretty easy to do!

1) First, fill a clear glass with room temperature water.

2) Get some clean hair strands, and put them in the water. These can be hairs from detangling, but the important thing is that they are clean. If they have product in them, you won't get an accurate result. So wash the strands with soap if you have to; you want an accurate result.

3) Let the strands air dry by placing them on a tissue, leaving them to dry naturally.

4) When dry, place them on the water and watch them for 2–5 minutes.

WHAT THE RESULTS MEAN

> If the hair sinks immediately, then it has high porosity because it absorbed the water and sank quickly.

> If it floats, then it has low porosity because it didn't absorb water well.

> If it sinks slowly, then it has normal porosity.

IMPLICATIONS

High porosity

High porosity hair benefits from heavier products and deep conditioning. My daughter has high porosity hair, but that means that it can lose moisture just as quickly as it gains it. If you have a similar problem, then I advise the following:

> Use coconut oil as a pre-shampoo to help reduce the amount by which the hair swells when wet and fortifies the protein in the hair strands.

> Use conditioners that contain a hydrolysed protein to help strengthen the hair.

> Use the LOC method when moisturizing and use a heavy cream or butter to seal the moisture in. If the case is extreme, you can consider using a product with an occlusive agent, such as mineral oil, to seal the moisture in place until the next wash.

Low porosity

Low porosity hair is often resistant to moisture, and when washing, it will take longer for the hair to get fully wet. I advise the following:

> When conditioning the hair, use a warm towel over a shower cap to encourage open cuticles so the benefits can be absorbed. If your child is old enough, consider using a hooded dryer for maximum benefit.

> When sealing the hair, use lighter oils such as grapeseed or jojoba.

> Try co-washing instead of shampooing to keep the hair as hydrated as possible.

> Try to keep the hair free of product build-up, as this can seal any moisture from being absorbed into the hair. Try to incorporate a cleansing shampoo or treatment into your regime once a month to keep the hair build-up free.

Normal porosity

Normal hair porosity hair is in optimum health. If this is your hair porosity, the only thing you need to do is adhere to the regime you are on, as it's working for you. Just keep up the good work! Remember to:

> Wash and deep condition weekly.

> Moisturize and seal when needed.

> Use protective styles the majority of the time.

HAIR THICKNESS

As we learned previously, the thickness of your daughter's actual strands can tell you more about the strength of her hair, while also revealing the requirements for any hair products.

HOW TO TEST HAIR THICKNESS

There isn't an easy or fast way to do this as with hair porosity, but here is a generally good way to determine hair thickness:

1) Obtain a few shed hairs when detangling.

2) Hold the hair up to the light and evaluate. If the hair is so thin that it's hard to see, then the conclusion can be made that your daughter has thin/skinny hair. If the hair is thick and clearly visible, then we can assume she has thick/ fatter hair.

IMPLICATIONS

Thin strands

If your daughter has thin strands, then know that her hair is likely to be more delicate. It will need more care in order for it to retain length (if that is your goal).

Make sure you:

> Use quality seamless hair tools.

> Use extra care when handling to reduce breakage.

> Try low-manipulation styles.

> Limit the use of brushes.

> Incorporate a conditioner with protein to help strengthen the hair and reduce breakage.

> Trim the ends if they are split or have single strand knots.

THICK STRANDS

Generally, thick strands are the stronger of the two, but that doesn't mean you can throw all caution to the wind. You must be sure to maintain a healthy hair care regime consistently.

Make sure you:

> Use heavier oils when sealing (such as castor oil) to hold the moisture in the hair.

> Don't assume the hair is strong enough for fine combs. It isn't. Stick to quality, seamless wide-tooth combs.

> Keep up your healthy hair care plan consistently.

NEXT STEPS

Relevant to toddlers and children, figuring out hair thickness and porosity is foundational to the techniques in the upcoming chapters. I will also make product and ingredient recommendations based on these results to eliminate any need for guessing games.

TOP INGREDIENTS TO LOOK FOR

Before we move onto more specific information on what products will work best for **your** daughter's hair in the 'Techniques' chapters, let's look at ingredients that are generally beneficial for hair.

These are common ingredients that you absolutely should be putting in your daughter's hair:

Water

Water is the basis for all life. It is the basis of sustenance and of cleansing. For hair, the same is true. Any moisturizer that doesn't list water as the first ingredient should not be considered. Just as our bodies get dehydrated, so does our hair. Both body and hair need water, and it is the basis for any potential for health. It's the ultimate moisturizer and contains molecules that are small enough to penetrate the hair shaft while also quenching the hair's thirst.

Shea butter

Produced from the Shea-Karite tree nut found in East and West Africa, unrefined shea butter has been referred to as 'mother nature's conditioner.' Its main components are essential fatty acids, including stearic, oleic and linoleic acids, vitamins E and D and pro-vitamin A. These provide super conditioning benefits to the hair.

Shea butter soothes irritated skin and the scalp, seals moisture into the hair, and adds sheen and creating softness for the hair. It also has antioxidant properties that can prevent damage from UV radiation. In short—it is a super food for hair!

Coconut oil

Obtained from mature fruits of coconut trees, some suggest that it was the first plant oil ever used by humanity. Solid at room temperature and composed of over 90% essential fatty acids, it includes lauric, myristic, caprylic, oleic and linoleic acids along with vitamin E, which condition, add lustre and provide sheen for the hair.

Its benefits include preventing hydral fatigue, fortifying hair by reducing protein loss, penetrating the hair for absorption and conditioning from within the hair. It's no surprise, then, that it has been touted as nature's best hair conditioner.

Aloe vera

Aloe vera juice and gel are obtained from the inner leaf of the plant and have been used for cosmetic, medicinal and health purposes for centuries because of their perceived healing capabilities. Aloe Vera contains antioxidants, antibiotics and antifungals. Its vitamins and minerals include folic acid, vitamins A, B1, B2, B6, C and E and amino acids. Aloe Vera is a humectant and is known to deliver moisture directly into the hair shaft.

It's possible to use both the gel and juice in hair and the benefits include nourishing and moisturizing, promoting hair growth, reducing dandruff and preventing hair loss.

Vegetable glycerin

Often a by-product of soap making, where palm, soy or coconut plant oils have been used, vegetable glycerin is a humectant and is often found in moisturizing sprays and leave-in conditioners.

Vegetable glycerin is a humectant and is used widely in hair and beauty products for its abilities to attract moisture to the hair and skin. The main benefits of glycerin are that it leaves the hair deeply moisturized. It also adds softness and pliability, making the hair easier to comb.

Jojoba oil

Jojoba oil is obtained from the seeds of the jojoba shrubs native to Arizona, California and Mexico, and has long been used as a carrier for essential oils. It's very high in vitamin E and also contains vitamins A, B1, B2 and B6. It contains essential fatty acids, including myristic acid and plant wax.

It's especially great with hair because it closely resembles hair's natural oil, sebum, and is readily accepted by the scalp and hair. It has anti-bacterial properties, which may help ease dandruff. It acts as an emollient, increasing pliability, shine, elasticity and softness of the hair.

Extra virgin olive oil

Not to be confused with regular olive oil, extra virgin olive oil is cold pressed from whole olives and is commonly used in cooking and cosmetics. Virgin means the oil was produced by mechanical means only, with no chemical treatment, and this makes it the grade that is most beneficial for hair.

Extra virgin olive oil is high in mono-unsaturated fatty acids and vitamins A and E. It is rich in anti-oxidants, which promote a healthy scalp and in turn healthy hair growth. Olive oil can clear up a dry scalp, boost shine, seal moisture and gradually increase tensile strength in hair.

Rosemary essential oil

Rosemary oil is an essential oil, so it is highly concentrated and will normally be used with a carrier oil to make it safer for skin and hair. Rosemary has long been associated with food, but today the oil is known for its antioxidant and antimicrobial properties.

Increasing scientific evidence has revealed that it's great for hair and can boost hair growth. It's also great for soothing a dry, irritated and itchy scalp while treating dandruff.

Avocado oil

Extra virgin avocado oil is extracted from the flesh of avocadoes by cold pressing. It's a dark green oil, rich in vitamins and minerals, including vitamins A, B1, B2 and B5. It also contains amino acids, magnesium and folic acid and essential fatty acids, which are all beneficial for healthy hair and scalp.

It's especially high in oleic acid, which closely resembles human sebum and is both moisturizing and regenerating. Its molecular structure means it can be absorbed by the skin and hair and is able to support and strengthen the hair fibre from within. It also nourishes, protects and unclogs hair follicles.

Castor oil

Castor oil is obtained from pressing the seeds of the castor oil plant and has a long history of being used in beauty treatments and products.

It's a pale yellow, heavy, and thick oil that is high in omega 6 and 9 essential fatty acids, vitamin E, minerals and proteins that are beneficial for the hair and scalp. It has long been thought that castor oil encourages hair growth, as it has a high concentration of ricinoleic acid, which helps increase blood flow to the scalp, which can encourage hair growth. It's great for hair because it is a natural humectant and will attract moisture from the environment into hair strands. It also locks in moisture well and adds shine and lustre.

Hydrolysed proteins

Hair is primarily made up of a protein called keratin, and by using hydrolysed proteins in our hair products, it's possible to fortify this keratin and strengthen the hair.

Hydrolysed proteins are proteins that have been broken down into smaller units that can be absorbed by the hair. The most common types you will see are hydrolysed wheat, silk, soy and keratin. They all help strengthen, moisturize, increase shine and smooth the hair.

Panthenol

Panthenol is a popular ingredient in hair and beauty products because it is a high performing humectant and helps the hair and skin retain moisture. It's derived from vitamin B5, which is an essential vitamin found in every living cell in the body.

Panthenol is known as a 'hair nourisher', and deeply penetrates the cuticles of hair. Its benefits include strengthening and moisturizing hair, adding sheen and lustre and producing more flexible and generally healthier hair.

So there you have it! Now you know what to avoid and what to look for, which will greatly help your daughter on her healthy hair journey! Do not forget: as we go through each technique, I will add product and ingredient recommendations for fine or thick and low, medium or high hair porosity types to help you in your product selection. But before we get there, we must first discuss the tools you will need on your healthy hair journey.

CHAPTER 10 TOOLS

Not all hair tools are created equally, and it's important that we select high quality appliances that don't snag, catch or snap the hair.

If we find a tool that causes damage to the hair, we must absolutely stop using it and find something else!

I advise that you have the following in your hair care arsenal:

QUALITY WIDE TOOTH COMB

Select a high quality, seamless comb to reduce snags.

SOFT BOAR BRISTLE BRUSH

Make sure the brush is 100% boar bristle and not synthetic. Buy the softest option.

SMALL HAIR BANDS (NOT ELASTIC)

ROUND CLIPS

For styling into bunches and buns.

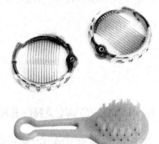

BABY HAIRBRUSH

BABY COMB

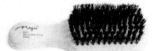

RAT-TAIL COMB (FOR PARTING)

Choose a comb with a metal tail to make parting easier.

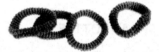

OUCHLESS HAIRBANDS

Good quality cotton hairbands used primarily to band the hair to dry it, stretched.

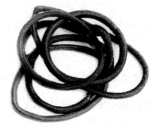

BUTTERFLY CLIPS

For sectioning hair when styling.

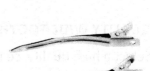

DUCK-BILL CLIPS

For sectioning hair when styling.

SPRAY BOTTLE X 3

For pre-shampoo mix, moisturizer mix (if homemade) and one spare!

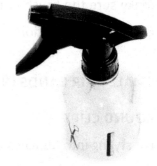

MIXING BOWL AND BRUSH

To mix and enhance conditioner, when required.

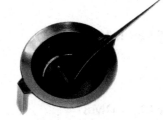

HAIR DRYER (WITH OPTIONAL CONCENTRATOR AND DIFFUSOR)

For tension method blow-drying.

TOOTHBRUSH

For baby hair styling.

PLASTIC SHOWER CAP

To cover head when conditioning.

SATIN CAP (OPTIONAL)

To protect the hair at night.

SATIN PILLOW CASE (OPTIONAL)

To protect the hair at night.

HEATED CONDITIONING CAP (OPTIONAL)

For use with older children to help conditioner process.

CHAPTER 11 TECHNIQUES

OUR AIM

As with anything in life, there are right and wrong ways to do things. Hair care is no different. In order to get the best results, the correct hair care practices have to be used at all times in order to avoid our enemy: breakage.

We need to combine theory with practice to get the best results, and in the following chapters you will learn the best hair care practices for optimum hair health.

Before we get to practice, we first have to lay down some house rules. These have to be upheld throughout the journey of optimizing your daughter's hair.

THE HOUSE RULES

The overarching rule: Any type of hair breakage is a no-no

Hair breaking is our number one enemy and we can't be nonchalant about it, even if it's only a small amount. Do not ignore what may very well be a difficult-to-reverse snowball effect!

If we see broken hairs, then we must pay immediate attention. Don't brush it off and think it will go away on its own. It will only get worse, and we want to avoid worse.

Tending to your daughter's hair requires a bit of detective work. Not only should hair breakage be identified but the reasons *why* the breakage is occurring need to be specified.

Sources of hair damage

There are a wide range of causes that spur broken hair, and some are due to medical conditions. We won't go into these conditions. Rather, we will examine what I have come to find as *self-inflicted* broken hair.

Below is a list of the most common sources of hair breakage:

> Lack of moisture/Dryness
> Force when combing
> Chemical processing
> Thermal styling
> Incorrect tools and product usage

Which brings us nicely along to the house rules that uphold our overarching rule!

RULE NUMBER 1 – KEEP THE HAIR MOISTURIZED

This one is simple: hair that is dry and brittle is prone to breakage. Overcome this by aiming to keep hair moisture levels optimized consistently.

RULE NUMBER 2 – BE GENTLE WITH HAIR

No heavy handedness. If you are hearing snapping when doing hair, then you are using too much force; it's your very own hand that is causing the breakage. Be gentle rather than abusive, use quality tools, and remember to treat hair with consideration and care. Give it love!

RULE NUMBER 3 – AVOID CHEMICALLY TREATING HAIR

Chemical treatment, relaxers and hair dyes can weaken hair and lead to damage. Avoid this by keeping the hair natural so it can be stronger and more resilient.

RULE NUMBER 4 – DON'T USE HEAT OFTEN

Regular direct heat usage from blow-dryers or flat irons can deplete the hair of moisture. Use direct heat with caution and sparingly.

RULE NUMBER 5 – USE THE CORRECT TOOLS AND PRODUCTS

Make sure you are using the correct tools when doing hair. Avoid fine-tooth combs and brushes and use your hands to detangle the hair as much as possible. Also make sure the products you are using are suitable and meet your requirements.

BONUS RULE

RULE NUMBER 6 – **STEPPING OFF THE GAS IS A NO-NO**

When it works, stay with it. Never give up on a good thing.

Imagine you have achieved your objective. Your daughter's hair is beautiful and healthy.

You might think that now's a good time to sit back, relax and take it easy. But that is not the case. Don't step off the gas with the hair care routine now, or ever, if it's working for you. What took so long to reach and maintain can easily disappear with negligence. It's funny, isn't it, how we can often look at an amazing result and overlook the effort required to achieve it.

People often look at my daughter's hair and say, "Well, she has long hair naturally," or the classic, "She's got great hair. You don't need to do all that much to it," without realizing that her hair is the way it is *because* of my efforts, not the other way around. The way I nurture it gets results. If I didn't take care of her hair the way I do, it wouldn't even be half the length it is because her hair is extremely dry naturally.

So think of it this way. A healthy hair care regime is for life...not just until you get the length you want!

Those are the house rules! Now we can look at the best practice techniques in the following chapters.

CHAPTER 12   THE PRE-SHAMPOO

TECHNIQUE 1: BEFORE YOU WASH HER HAIR, GIVE HER THE PRE-SHAMPOO TREATMENT

It's generally thought that hair washing is the starting point in the hair care cycle. The perception is that it starts everything off and that conditioning and styling follow. This perception is built upon the idea that shampooing refreshes the hair and gets it ready for another action of styling.

The majority of women will jump straight in and wash hair after taking it out of its previous style. But when creating a healthy hair care regime, there are a few additional steps we need to take before we wash for maximum health benefits.

FUNCTION OF THE PRE-SHAMPOO TREATMENT

The functions of a pre-shampoo treatment are to (a) coat the hair before washing so the shampoo doesn't strip the natural oils from the hair, (b) coat the hair to reduce hydral fatigue and (c) function as a conditioning treatment.

Frequency

Before every wash!

Method

It's very easy to do on children's hair, and there are two main ways to do it.

1) When taking hair out of its previous style, coat hands in oil to increase manageability and reduce friction and breakage. Once all the hair is loose, apply a generous amount of oil to hair and scalp, twist into 6 sections and let the oil sit with a plastic cap for as long as you can before washing.

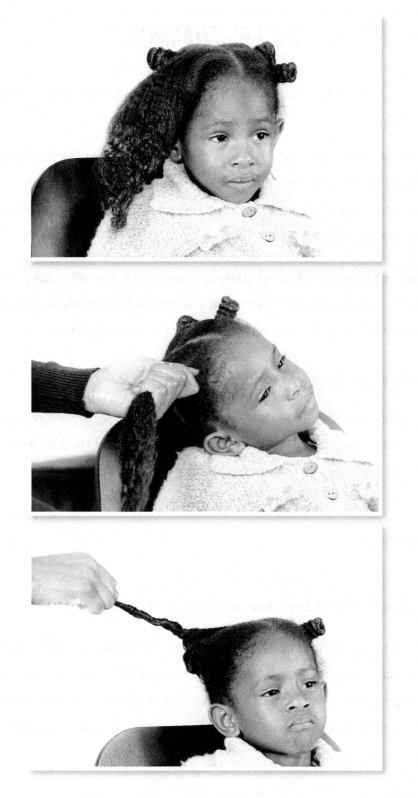

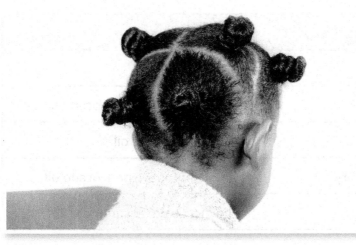

2) You can also use the oil for a hot oil treatment prior to washing. To do this, loosen the hair with oil as described above, but before applying the oil directly to the hair warm it up on the stove or in the microwave to a tolerable temperature. Then proceed to apply it to the hair, twist into 6 sections and cover with a plastic cap (optional).

3) You can also enhance the oil with an essential oil for added benefits. To do this, get a mixing bowl and add 4 tablespoons of the oil of your choice along with 5 drops of rosemary, peppermint or tea tree oil. It can be applied either cold or warm to the scalp and hair and will cleanse for a healthy scalp while stimulating for healthy hair growth.

RECOMENDATIONS

If your daughter has...	Use (optional)
Fine hair	Coconut oil
Thick hair	Coconut, olive or avocado oil
Low porosity	Warm coconut oil
Medium porosity	Coconut, olive or avocado oil
High porosity	Avocado oil, coconut oil

For a scalp treatment, add 3–5 drop of rosemary, tea tree or peppermint oil to the oil before applying to the scalp.

CHAPTER 13 DETANGLING

TECHNIQUE 2: BEFORE WASHING, PROPERLY DETANGLE THE HAIR

Function

Now, the function of detangling is pretty self-explanatory. It's the process by which we unravel the hair, so it's possible to comb through the hair smoothly and without snags. We really, really, really, really don't like tangles. And we really want to get them out of the hair with little to no breakage.

We want to remove all the tangles from the hair *before* washing it because water and tangles can result in knotted and matted hair, which can be difficult to remove without breakage.

Frequency

Your daughter's hair will need to be detangled before washing, once a week. It may also be necessary to do it again before styling. But ideally, we only want a comb to go through the hair once a week or twice at the absolute maximum.

Method (3 inches and longer)

So to detangle the hair, this is what I recommend:

1) First, we need to break the hair down into four to six sections. We are going to part it down the middle from forehead to nape and then across the centre from ear to ear. We can then clip each section with a butterfly clip or put it into bantu knots.

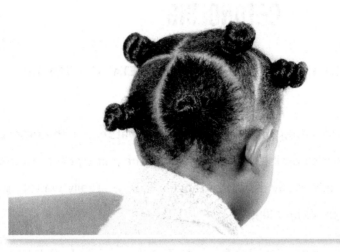

2) Then we're going to wet the hair using a spray bottle and warm water, section by section. Then we can apply a generous amount of instant conditioner to the mid-lengths to the ends of the hair, per section.

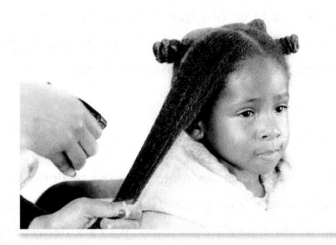

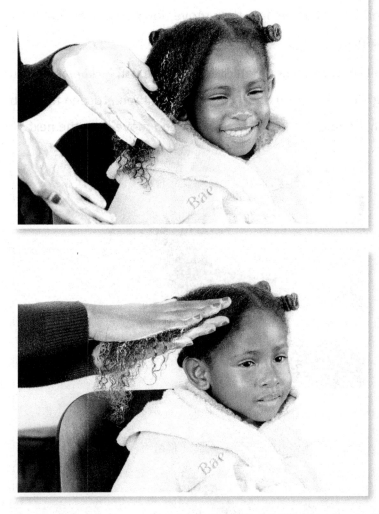

An instant conditioner is a non-penetrating, generally cheap conditioner. It's something you can pick up in your supermarket that will make the hair very slippery and easy to work with.

3) Then we can start to detangle the hair.

To do this, first we're going to start with our hands and not the comb, concentrating on the ends of the hair. You never detangle from the roots because it will lead to breakage. Always the ends of the hair first!

So taking your first section, you will start at the ends and remove the tangles by hand from that section, then move down 2" and repeat until you reach the scalp.

You will know the hair is detangled because you will be able to run your fingers through it smoothly in one stroke. You can then proceed to comb through that section, braid it in a loose single plait, and move onto the next.

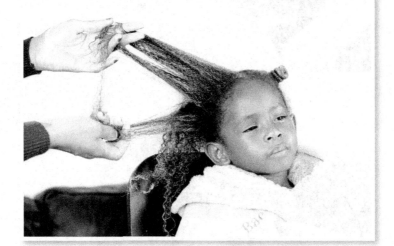

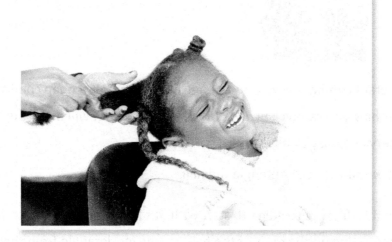

DETANGLING HAIR IN BABIES

Detangling a baby's hair is a pretty straightforward and easy process and, in fact, I would say that until the hair is around 3", there shouldn't be too much of a need to have a focused detangling session. But there is no hard and fast rule on this, so you will have to be the judge on what is best for your baby's hair.

If you find that the hair is prone to tangling and find that after washing, it's difficult to finger detangle or comb, then carry out the detangling technique for toddlers as detailed above.

Generally for babies, I would suggest to

1) Coat the hair in olive oil,
2) Finger detangle
3) Gently comb through starting at the ends with a baby comb or baby brush (you won't need to put it in plaits to wash it).

TOP TIP

As the hair starts to get curlier or more afro in texture, it's likely to tangle more. You're going to need to factor in detangling in your daughter's hair care regime. If you don't, it will lead to mats, knots and breakage.

RECOMMENDATIONS

If your daughter has...	Use (optional)
Fine hair	Conditioner containing silicones for added slip
Thick hair	Conditioner containing silicones for added slip, followed by a coating of oil of your choice
Low porosity	Conditioner containing silicones for added slip
Medium porosity	Conditioner containing silicones for added slip
High porosity	Conditioner containing silicones for added slip, followed by a coating of an oil of your choice

When dealing with fidgety children, I advocate using a conditioner with silicones for this step, because it will greatly increase manageability and slip and reduce tangles and breakage. We have had great success using Herbal Essences' *Hello Hydration* conditioner for this step.

CHAPTER 14 WASHING

TECHNIQUE 3: WASHING YOUR DAUGHTER'S HAIR

Washing hair may seem like a no brainer. It seems so simple and straightforward, but believe it or not, there are right and wrong ways to wash your daughter's hair.

Function

The primary function of washing the hair is to clean the scalp and to remove any dirt, debris or product build-up. Our aim is to create a healthy and clean environment in which hair can grow healthily.

It's not to say that the ends of the hair won't get clean also, but our focus is the scalp. The rest of the hair will get clean as the shampoo is rinsed and travels down the hair strands.

No rubbing in circles

I'm sure we have all see the TV adverts: a woman is in the shower, her hair is piled up on top of her head, she is using a generous amount of shampoo and she is rubbing her hair round and round in circles. This common image comes to mind when people think of hair washing.

For obvious reasons, the standing up in the shower bit won't work for children's hair! But rubbing the shampoo on in circular motions is something a lot of us do without realizing, and this doesn't work well for afro hair because it causes tangles.

Frequency

This may come as a shock to some people, but you only need to shampoo the hair **once** and not repeat it 2-3 times, as you may have been told.

We need to remember that we are dealing with children's hair here, and they are not likely to have gel, hairspray or heavy products in their hair, so shampooing it once will suffice for keeping the scalp and hair adequately clean. Anything more than this can cause the shampoo to strip the hair of its natural oils, which can result in dryness and, in turn, breakage.

I would recommend that you wash your daughter's hair at least once a week. I know, I know, to some of us that can seem like a lot, but hear me out on this one. When we wash and condition the hair, we are actually reintroducing moisture into the hair and this helps to keep the hair hydrated and can improve the overall condition of the hair.

WASHING IN STYLES

Depending on your child's hair length, it may also be possible to wash the hair whilst it is in a style.

In my experience, this works well for certain styles, such as individual braids or individual twists, and not so well in others, like cornrows. But I would recommend doing this only once before removing them and washing as normal the following week.

Methods

Now, the best method for washing the hair will obviously change depending on the age of the child and the length of the hair. If you're dealing with a baby, the best time to wash their hair is during or just before bath time. If a toddler, then bath time is still an option, but you can also have designated hair-washing time.

WASHING BABIES HAIR (UNDER 3")

Washing babies' hair can be daunting at first, especially when they are tiny and appear to be so delicate! But it is possible to do it successfully. Here's how:

1) Firstly, you should have everything you need to hand to make it as easy as possible for yourself.

   You will need:

   > 2 towels
   > 2 jugs of lukewarm water
   > Shampoo

2) Then, hold the baby over the bath and use a jug of clean, lukewarm water to fully saturate their hair. Make sure the water doesn't have any soaps in it. Hence, using bath water is not advised. You just want plain, lukewarm water.

3) Then you can shampoo the hair. I would recommend getting the shampoo onto the pads of your fingertips on one hand and gently smoothing it into the hair, using a non-circular motion, making sure you get all areas of the hair, the front and the back.

4) Then you're going to proceed to rinse it out, again using a jug of clean, lukewarm water, and repeat if necessary until all the shampoo is gone.

WASHING TODDLERS' OR YOUNG CHILDREN'S HAIR

It might not continue to be practical to wash your young child's hair in the bath, especially when they start learning to wriggle and kick.

You can wash it at the kitchen sink, if you have a space next to your sink where they are able to lie down and lean their head back under the tap. Or you can wash it whilst they are on your lap, with their head back over the bath (my fave!).

HOW TO DO THE BATH METHOD

1) To do this, you need a small chair; put this parallel to the bath, sit down, and you will be adjacent to the bath. You should be sitting next to the bath, facing

in the same direction as you would be if you were sitting in it. Roll up a towel and put it on the edge of the bath as in pic.

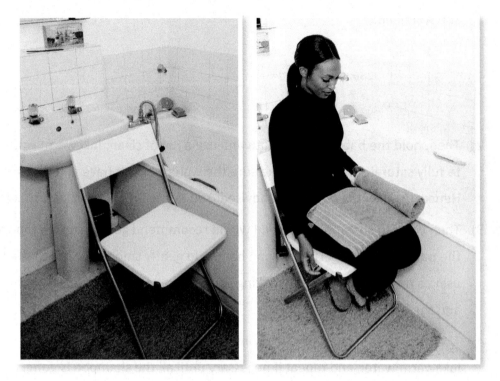

2) Then put your little one on your lap with their back to the bath. Lean them back, face up, and rest the back of their neck on the rolled up towel. Their head should be over the bath.

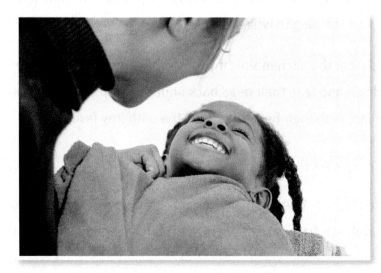

3) Then use the shower and wash the hair; it should be a similar result to having it washed in the salon. Ideally, you want to use one hand to hold the shower and the other to massage the scalp.

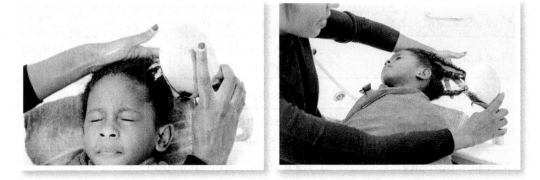

This method has been the most successful way I have washed Bae's hair, and I tried a few different techniques! Prior to this, we were fighting at wash time. I was trying to physically hold her over the sink, but she would squirm and wriggle about and I couldn't hold her. This way we both enjoy because it enables her to feel calm, and it enables me to get the job done with no stress.

TOP TIP

I'd advise that for hair over 3", you wash it in 4-6 single plaits as detailed in technique 2 to minimize tangling when washing.

When you have washed the hair, wring it out gently by hand, then towel blot it gently and get ready to condition the hair.

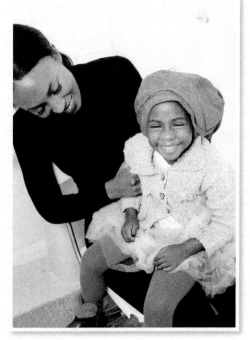

RECOMMENDATIONS

Always aim for a moisturizing shampoo! If the shampoo you are using leaves the hair feeling stripped, try adding a teaspoon of olive or avocado oil to it.

If your daughter has...	Use (optional)
Fine hair	A sulfate-free shampoo, possibly containing proteins
Thick hair	A sulfate-free shampoo
Low porosity	A sulfate-free shampoo, warmer water to open the hair follicles.
Medium porosity	A sulfate-free shampoo
High porosity	A sulfate-free shampoo, containing humectants

CHAPTER 15 CONDITIONING

TECHNIQUE 4: CONDITIONING YOUR DAUGHTER'S HAIR

Function

Conditioning the hair is a cornerstone in any healthy hair care regime. The aim with conditioning is either to maintain or improve the current condition of the hair by raising its moisture and/or protein levels.

There are different types of conditioners that you will use in your daughter's healthy hair regime. You will use an instant conditioner when detangling and a deep conditioner for regular treatment.

An instant conditioner is something that you can pick up in your local supermarket. It's a conditioner that doesn't have many or any ingredients that are able to penetrate into the hair, but instead it will coat the hair and make the hair feel very soft, making it slippery and manageable. It's the slip that we are looking for with an instant conditioner. It reduces tension when detangling, which reduces hair breakage.

A deep conditioner, on the other hand, is a conditioner that's designed to penetrate into the hair shaft and strengthen it from the inside out. There are two types of deep conditioner: moisture-based and protein-based.

Frequency

You need to condition the hair at least once a week with a moisturizing conditioner. Protein conditioners are optional, depending on the hair's needs. You may or may not use instant conditioners, depending on how long the hair is and how difficult it is to detangle.

It's not essential to use heat on a child's hair to condition it, unless we are dealing with low porosity hair. In all other circumstances, I recommend leaving the conditioner on for 10 minutes, covered by a plastic cap with a woolly hat or towel on top.

It's important not to let your child out of your sight if you choose to put a plastic cap on them because of possible suffocation or choking risks that come immediately with any plastic bag or cap. But I have found that with my daughter, the cap plus woolly hat causes her head to warm up, which in turn helps the conditioner to penetrate her hair.

Method

The best way to condition the hair, I have found, is when the hair is damp. Some people will condition dry hair and others will condition when the hair is soaking wet, but in my experience, I recommend conditioning damp, towel-dried hair.

THE BEST METHOD FOR CONDITIONING HAIR 3" AND LONGER

1) I recommend towel-blotting your daughter's hair and sitting her on your lap. To avoid getting cold, it is a good idea to wrap a towel around her or put on her dressing gown if she has one.

    If her hair is over 3", then it is likely you will have washed the hair in plaits. If not, please see the section below on conditioning baby hair.

2) Start with a section and gently un-plait it and run your fingers through it. It should still be tangle-free; towel-blot it and put a generous amount of conditioner in your hands, rub them together and

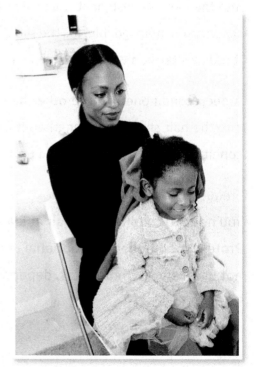

smooth it through that section of hair, concentrating from the mid lengths to ends. Finger comb the conditioner through the hair and re-plait. Then move onto the next section and repeat until you have done all sections.

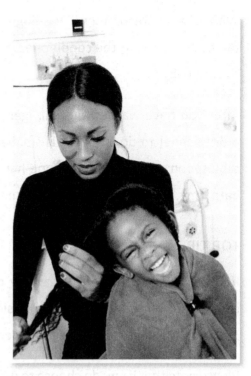

If you have not washed the hair in plaits or experience some tangling when finger combing, then you will need to go through the detangling process on each section as you go.

DON'T FORGET TO CONDITION THE HAIRLINE

Although hair conditioner focuses on the mid lengths to the ends of the hair, there is one exception when you will put it onto the scalp and that is in the hairline.

For infants, the hair in the hairline is often the most delicate and needs conditioner too! The hairline is likely where your daughter is going to have shorter hair and we ultimately want it to grow and catch up to the rest of her hair, so we do need to make sure that it is conditioned as well.

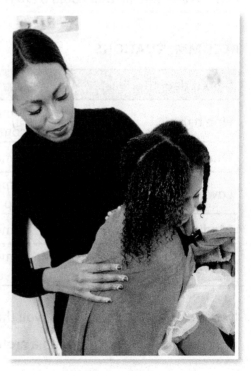

CONDITIONING BABIES' HAIR

The method for conditioning baby's hair is slightly different from young children's hair because infants generally have a lot less hair and will not have designated hair wash time.

With a baby, I recommend washing and conditioning their hair as soon as they get in the bath. That way, the conditioner gets to spend time in the hair as you wash the rest of your baby.

After you have washed the hair, gently towel-blot it (you might find it useful to use a dry flannel to do this as it is smaller and easier to work with). Then apply about a tablespoon of conditioner to one hand and smooth it through the hair. At the end of bath time, rinse the conditioner from the hair.

TOP TIP

If your child suffers from extremely dry hair, then my advice is to not wash all the conditioner out of her hair when rinsing it. I would advise you aim to wash about 50% of it out and leave the rest in for added hydration.

Please note that if you do choose to do this, it is best to use organic and natural products with no ingredients that could be harmful or irritating for your baby.

RECOMMENDATIONS

If your daughter has...	Use (optional)
Fine hair	A moisturizing deep conditioner, possibly containing hydrolysed proteins or silk amino acids
Thick hair	A moisturizing deep conditioner
Low porosity	A moisturizing deep conditioner used with shower cap and towel
Medium porosity	A moisturizing deep conditioner
High porosity	A moisturizing deep conditioner, combined with olive or avocado oil

If your daughter has fine hair or you think she may have a need for protein conditioning, then do this once a month with a protein rich conditioner

CHAPTER 16 PRODUCT LAYERING

TECHNIQUE 5: PRODUCT LAYERING FOR MAXIMUM MOISTURE RETENTION

Function

The correct layering of products is another fundamental aspect to a healthy hair care regime. It's not sufficient to rely on just one product to meet all of your requirements, as it most likely won't. You need a good product combination to get maximum benefits, and when you find a product combo your daughter's hair loves, you will hit your stride!

There are different ways to layer products, but I'm only going to talk about two that have worked well for us. The moisture and seal method and the liquid oil cream (LOC) method.

Frequency

You need to layer products into her hair after every wash, so this will be weekly.

You may also layer products daily (see daily maintenance).

THE LOC METHOD

The L-O-C or the Liquid-Oil-Cream method is a great way to keep the hair hydrated. We've had tremendous success with this method, and for extreme dry hair it works wonders in keeping hair hydrated and soft.

The basic premise of this method is straightforward and makes practical sense.

Step 1 – Apply a water-based moisturizer to the hair.

Step 2 – Apply oil to the hair.

Step 3 – Apply a cream to the hair.

This method is great for use just after washing the hair to seal as much moisture into the hair as is possible! After washing, towel-blot the hair so it is damp and not soaking wet. I advise working in sections, so if you have washed in plaits, work section by section.

1) Even though your daughter's hair is still likely to be damp after washing, I would recommend that you still apply a water-based moisturizer or a leave-in conditioner as the first step. You won't need to apply a lot, and will concentrate on the mid lengths to ends.

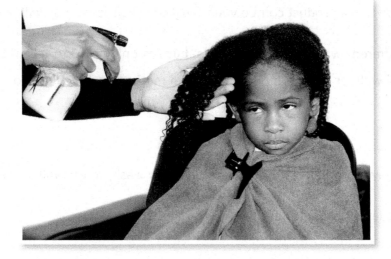

2) Then you move onto your oil and again smooth this through the mid lengths to ends. What oil you select will depend on your daughter's hair needs. Generally, the drier the hair, the thicker the oil. We have used coconut, olive and jojoba oil to much success. But I would advise you to try a few different ones and see what leaves your daughter's hair feeling the softest after it has dried.

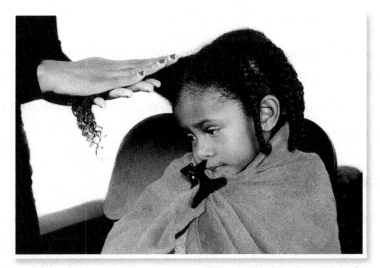

3) Then, the final layer is cream, and there are different ways of doing this. I would recommend you either use a specific hair moisturizing heavy cream, an organic conditioner or a hair butter.

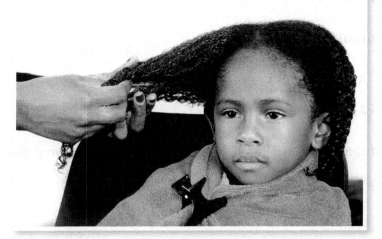

You will want to go through the hair section-by-section and put each one in two strand twists ready for styling when complete.

There are no set rules about what product you should use for each step because what works for one may not work for another. But experiment and find out what products work best for your daughter.

TOP TIP

A good indicator of a product working is how moisturized and soft the hair feels after it has dried with the products in it. For example, I just made a tweak in my daughter's products, and the hair feels significantly softer when it is dry now. The new products have become a staple in her regime.

THE MOISTURE AND SEAL METHOD

This is a fantastic method for daily maintenance of the hair and also after washing for hair that is not super dry. The basic thinking behind this method is that unless moisture is sealed into the hair, it will just evaporate. With this, we are trapping moisture in the hair.

It's similar to, but not as heavy duty as, the LOC method, and I have had great success with it on a daily basis.

It's so simple to do!

Step one – Apply a water-based moisturizer to the hair.

Step two – Apply oil.

It really is that simple. Again, there is no hard or fast rule as to what products you use. You need to figure out what works best for your daughter's hair.

TOP TIP

It's likely that as your child's hair grows and changes, its needs will change as well. There are no rules; it's up to you to figure out what her hair loves, and that will take some experimentation.

For both methods, towel-blot the hair so it is damp before applying the first layer. Hair is a bit like a sponge, so we need to get rid of the excess water in order for it to absorb more moisture.

RECOMMENDATIONS

If your daughter has...	Use (optional)
Fine hair	Moisture and seal, final seal being a cream containing proteins (e.g., cantu shea butter leave-in)
Thick hair	L.O.C.
Low porosity	L.O.C. liquid layer should contain water and humectants. Cream should be a hair butter.
Medium porosity	Moisture and seal or L.O.C.
High porosity	L.O.C., final layer being a hair butter, possibly one containing a polar oil to hold in moisture

CHAPTER 17 DRYING

TECHNIQUE 6: DRYING HER HAIR

The next technique we're going to talk about is drying the hair, which is the next step after product layering.

As you recall, house rule number 4 advises against using heat often, so I'm not a great big advocate for blow-drying the hair often. I think it's okay to do it to check the length of the hair and for special occasions, but it's not something I recommend to do week in and week out. It will cause dryness.

So then the question comes, "How do I dry my daughter's hair on a regular basis?"

AIR-DRYING IS THE WAY

Letting the hair dry naturally through air-drying is the best way to dry natural hair. By doing it, the hair will retain as much moisture as possible, and there won't be the breakage or snapping that can come from blow-drying.

Function

The best way to see the benefits of air-drying is to compare it to blow-drying.

With blow-drying, you normally use a hot dryer with a comb attachment and go over the hair several times until it is dry. This is bad news for afro hair on several fronts. Firstly, the action of combing through the hair with the dryer is likely to snap the hair in its fragile places. Secondly, the hot air literally forces all the moisture that was in the strand of the hair out and can cause excessive dryness.

Frequency

You are going to want to air dry your daughter's hair 98% of the time. You can maybe think about blow-drying the hair up to twice a year, but no more.

Method

Now, what you're going to want to do after your child's hair has been washed, conditioned and has products applied is proceed straight to drying it. Don't wait around and let the hair air dry while loose and then take this step. Straight after the hair has had the products layered in is when you will want to do this, to minimize tangling.

Drying natural hair is ridiculously simple! You're just going to style it or band it and let it dry. This way the hair will dry and yet be moisturized at the same time!

STYLE FROM WET

If your daughter's hair is over 3", it's likely that you will have washed it in plaits. If not, then use a clip to keep the hair separated so you only have out what you will be working with.

Then go ahead and style her hair! It is super easy to work with damp hair; however, if you are doing the LOC method, please see the top tip below.

Ideal styles include cornrows, flat twists, single twists and plaits for hair over 3". For shorter hair, I advise loose single plaits or twists and then bunches or something similar when it dries.

TOP TIP

If you are doing the LOC method and are using natural hair butter, I would advise styling the hair and then applying the butter. This is because natural butters are heavy and can make it difficult to separate the hair for braiding.

BANDING

Another way to dry the hair is using the Banding Method, which is a way to stretch and elongate the hair as it dries. This makes the hair easier to style if you are not comfortable or confident with wet styling the hair. Banding is based on the African method of threading the hair. Threading is where hair is put into small sections and thread is wound around the hair to stretch the hair out as it dries.

I'd recommend it on hair longer than 5".

This is what you do.

1) It's likely the hair will be in 6 sections, so start with a section at the back. Check that the section of hair is detangled and then split that in half. In total, we are going for 8-12 sections when banding the hair. The number will depend on the length and thickness of the hair. Clip away the hair you are not presently banding.

2) To band the hair, start at the base and apply your first band just as you would if you were putting the hair into a ponytail. Then put another band in, around an inch down from the first one, then another an inch down from that one and so on, repeating down the length of the hair. Then repeat in each section until you have done all of the hair.

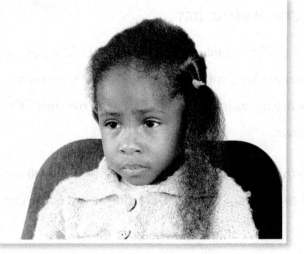

Hair will normally dry overnight in bands and be ready for styling the next day. Obviously the time it takes will differ depending on how many sections you do. Generally speaking, the more sections, the quicker it is to dry and the fewer sections, the longer it will take.

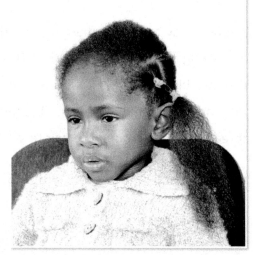

TOP TIP

I recommend using small, soft cotton bands for this; please see the 'Tools' chapter for details. NEVER use elastic bands.

BLOW-DRYING

There will be times when you need to blow dry your daughter's hair. And I recommend the tension method to reduce the amount of direct heat on the hair and the extent of manipulation.

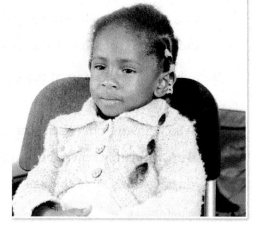

TENSION METHOD BLOW-DRY

After washing the hair, apply a leave-in product followed by a heat protector, which is essential when working with any type of direct heat on hair. Don't put oil on the hair prior to blow-drying, as it can cause the hair to overheat. Oils can be used after the hair has cooled down.

1) To do this method, you will need to work in small sections, so part the hair into small sections to work with, starting at the nape. Clip everything else away.

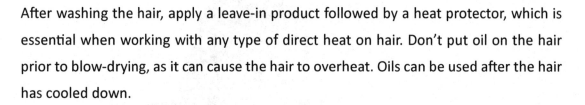

2) Using one hand to hold the hair dryer and the other to pull the hair taut, start at the base and direct the heat up and down the strands until they are dry.

3) Part another section and repeat the process until all the hair is dry.

TOP TIP

I recommend using a blow-dryer with a concentrator attachment and on a medium setting, because hot will be too much and cold will take too long!

RECOMMENDATIONS

If your daughter has...	Try
Fine hair	Styling from damp
Thick hair	Try banding
Low porosity	Styling from damp
Medium porosity	Banding or styling from damp
High porosity	Styling from damp with an extra layer of oil before styling

In all cases, limit the use of direct heat to no more than 2 times a year!

CHAPTER 18   PROTECTIVE STYLING

TECHNIQUE 7: STYLING TO PROTECT THE ENDS OF THE HAIR FROM BREAKAGE

Function

The function of protective styling is to literally protect the ends of the hair from breakage and retain as much length as the hair grows. We know short hair syndrome is caused by breakage; so protective styling is our antidote to that. Protective styles can also help the hair to retain moisture.

It's important to remember that the ends of the hair are its oldest parts. Like any other structure, the oldest parts generally tend to be the most vulnerable. And in the case of hair, the old ends of hair happen to be the most dry and delicate. They need special attention!

Frequency

Protective styles should be worn 90% of the time when your daughter's hair is long enough. These styles are a tremendous growth aide.

Method

Where the hair is long enough, the easiest protective styles are going to be cornrows, flat-twists, single twist or plaits.

Don't worry if you can't plait! We have tutorials coming up later on.

I recommend styles that keep the hair off the shoulders. We do not want the ends of the hair constantly rubbing on clothes and breaking.

There is a common issue in the natural community of growing hair past what's called "the shoulder length hump". That is, growing hair past the shoulders and down the back. It is notoriously difficult to grow afro hair past this hump if it is worn out because the hair will rest on the shoulders and will constantly rub, which can cause dryness and breakage in the ends, which will stop it retaining length.

PROTECTIVE STYLES IN BABIES

In babies, it is not so easy to do protective styles because the hair may not be long enough to braid, plait or twist. Focus on keeping the hair hydrated, and that may mean applying a moisturizer more frequently. You don't need to worry too much about protective styles until the hair is at a length that it can be braided or twisted. When the hair is long enough, put it in bunches and ponytails to offer it some protection.

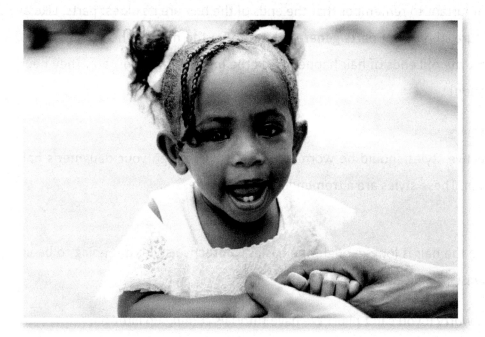

Bunches are a great protective style for babies.

RECOMMENDATIONS

If your daughter has...	Try
Fine hair	Avoid super small styles, as they will be difficult to remove. Try medium to large size braids and twists
Thick hair	Banding or styling from damp, small, medium or large braids and twists
Low porosity	Cornrows or flat twists from damp
Medium porosity	Banding or styling from damp, small, medium or large braids and twists
High porosity	Single twists/braids from damp

These are just basic suggestions. Feel free to experiment with your own hairstyles also!

CHAPTER 19 DAILY MAINTENANCE

TECHNIQUE 8: DAILY MAINTENANCE FOR OPTIMAL MOISTURE LEVELS

Function and frequency

The function of moisturizing is a simple one. We need to keep afro hair hydrated because it is the driest hair type. We can't rely on our hair to moisturize itself, so we must take action into our own hands. It's crucially important to maintain the moisture levels in your daughter's hair on a *consistent basis.*

It is something we need to do daily, and in some instances twice daily, morning and evening.

Hair conditions either need to be preserved or improved, and these benchmarks should be kept in mind to avoid it from going dry. No matter how much you water it, like a shrivelled up plant bringing dry hair back to nourished levels takes a lot of work and consistency.

Method

You can either use the LOC or Moisture & Seal method as your daily maintenance, depending on how dry the hair is and what the hair responds positively to.

You will start with your water-based moisturizer.

1) You will want to lightly mist the hair. There is no need to get it super damp.

2) Then follow with your oil or oil and cream.

It's pretty straightforward, and you can read how to do it in the Product layering chapter.

TOP TIP

You only need to use a small amount of each product. Definitely use less than you do on washday. Because you are doing it daily, I recommend about half a teaspoon of each product.

If you have determined that your daughter's hair needs two applications a day, then do one first thing in the morning and last thing before bedtime. If you are only doing one, do it before bedtime.

IMPORTANT! Don't over-moisturize or keep it in a constant state of dampness. The hair should feel dry before another round of moisturizer is applied

RECOMMENDATIONS

If your daughter has...	Try
Fine hair	Light moisturizer (e.g., water and aloe vera juice mixed), followed by light oil
Thick hair	Heavier moisturizer (e.g., S-Curl), followed by oil and cream
Low porosity	Light moisturizer (e.g., water and aloe vera juice mixed with added humectant), followed by light oil
Medium porosity	Light or heavy moisturizer (Moisture and seal or L.O.C.)
High porosity	Heavier moisturizer (e.g., S-Curl), followed by oil, then cream (L.O.C.)

CHAPTER 20 NIGHT TIME CARE

TECHNIQUE 9: **PROTECTING THE HAIR AT NIGHT**

Function and frequency

We spend a considerable amount of time asleep. The idea behind night-time hair care is to take advantage of this time and put it to use for hair health in a positive way. At night, hair moisture can be lost to pillows, sheets and blankets and we want to minimize this.

When we sleep on cotton, it actually sucks out the moisture from the hair, so we need to put some barriers in place to reduce this.

Method

There are two main ways to protect the hair at night.

1) Use a satin scarf or sleep cap

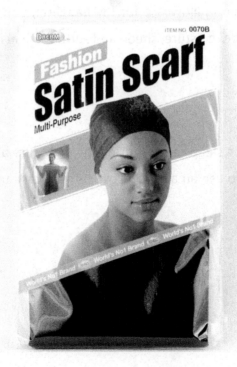

OR

2) Use a satin pillowcase

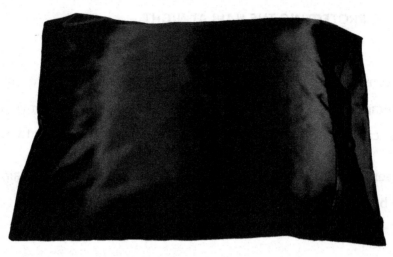

Satin is a great material because it doesn't draw as much moisture out of the hair as cotton does. It might seem like a gimmick, which is how I initially saw it, but it actually works!

I recently purchased a satin pillowcase for my daughter, and I can report that in the morning her hair had more moisture, sheen and softness than it had after sleeping with cotton sheets.

TOP TIP

If your child cannot keep a sleep cap on during the night, use a satin pillowcase! Even if they are not at the age to use an actual pillow, put the case underneath their head to protect the hair.

RECOMMENDATIONS

If your daughter has...	Try
Fine hair	Satin pillow case or satin sleep cap or scarf
Thick hair	Satin pillow case or satin sleep cap or scarf
Low porosity	Satin pillow case or satin sleep cap or scarf
Medium porosity	Satin pillow case or satin sleep cap or scarf
High porosity	Satin pillow case or satin sleep cap or scarf

So, now that you have reached the end of the techniques chapters, we will now move onto how to braid and plait.

CHAPTER 21   TWISTING AND FLAT-TWISTING

As a bonus for those of you not confident in twisting or flat twisting, I've included full instructions on how to do it!

Twisting is a great starting place for natural hair styling because it is super easy to do and to remove. Twists are versatile and work well for babies with delicate hair right through to older children with all hair types and textures.

In my experience, twists are a perfect style for toddlers because they allow the style to be adapted slightly from day to day. For example, one day they can be styled in a bun, the next bunches, the next half up and half down and so on and so forth.

An added bonus is that it is really easy to moisturize hair in twists, and you can really get to all of the hair with ease. Also, twists look fantastic when taken out for a twist out, which is a more defined curly look.

A routine I got into with my daughter is that she has single twist while at day care for the majority of the week, and for the weekend I take them out so she can have a twist out until I wash her hair again a few days later. I find it to be a great way for us both to really enjoy her hair.

CLASSIC TWO STRAND TWIST

This is a cute, quick and easy-to-do style that produces versatile results.

YOU WILL NEED:

Rat-tail comb for parting

Wide toothcomb for detangling

Butterfly clips for sectioning

Here's how you do it:

1) Part the section of hair to be twisted and clip everything else away. From your section, take 2 pieces of hair in equal size.

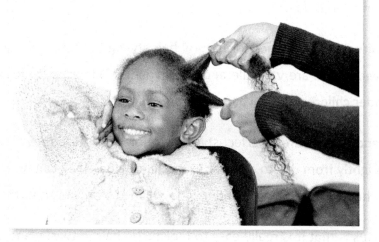

2) Hold each piece between your thumb and index finger on each hand.

3) Take the right section and put it under the left section and repeat. You are now twisting the hair!

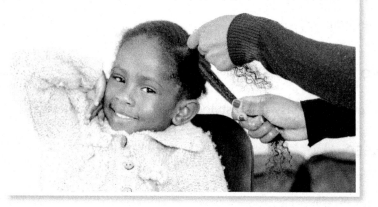

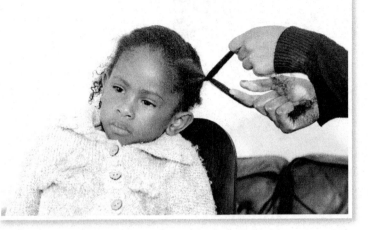

4) The twist should resemble a rope; continue down the length of the hair.

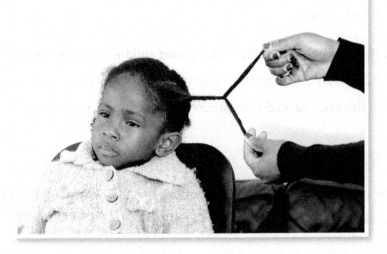

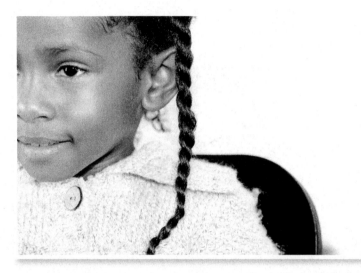

5) Part another section of hair and repeat until all the hair is twisted.

And it really is that simple!

Twists are perfect for babies, toddlers and young children and can be left in the hair for ideally a week, but can also stretch to two weeks. At night, twists should be worn in a loose bun with the ends tucked in to prevent them from losing too much moisture.

FLAT TWISTS

Flat twists are similar in appearance to cornrows, but they are much easier and faster to do. If you can twist hair, then you can do flat twists!

They are fantastic for highly textured hair because they keep the hair protected and stay in place for a standard 1–2 weeks. Similar to two-strand twists, they can be taken out for a twist out, a defined, natural, curly look.

YOU WILL NEED:

Rat-tail comb for parting

Wide tooth comb for detangling

Butterfly clips for sectioning

1) Larger flat twists are best for learning on, so start by parting the hair from front to back. Plan your first row, part it out, and clip everything else away.

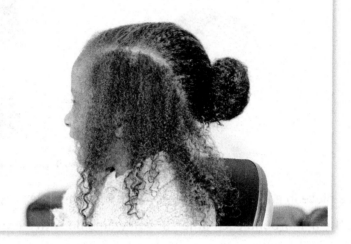

2) Make sure the hair to be twisted is detangled completely.

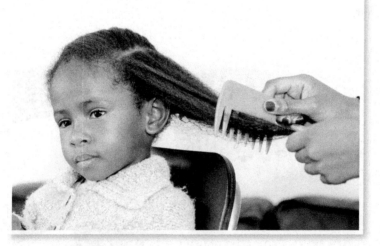

3) Position your child in front of you, and at the front of the row, start with a small section of hair divided into 2 equal-size pieces.

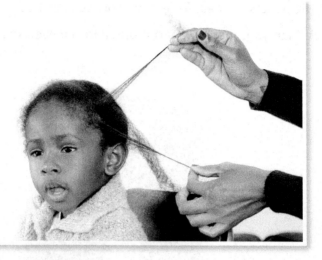

4) Hold a piece in each hand between you thumb and index finger and begin to twist the hair around each other, as you would do with a normal twist.

5) Start off by doing 1 rotation of a normal twist, but on the third rotation, as you go back, gently pick up more hair from the middle section to incorporate into the twist.

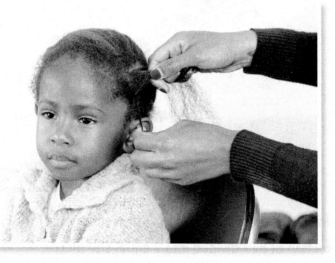

6) Continue until you reach the end of the row, and if the hair is long enough, continue down to the ends of the hair with a regular two-strand twist.

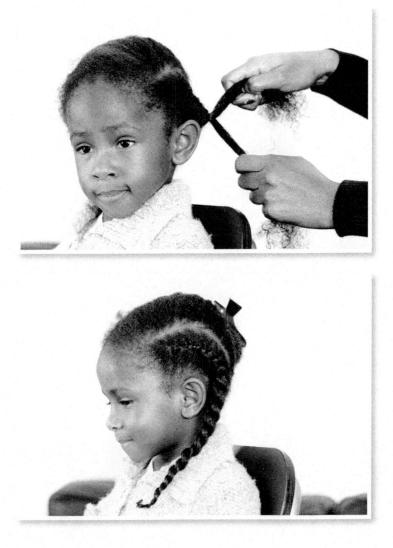

MORE FLAT TWIST STYLES

Flat twists are considerably easier to do than cornrows, and they work great for children. Although not as versatile as two-strand twists, they can still be styled into buns, bunches and other styles, but very intricate styles will require cornrows because they allow for more detail.

CHAPTER 22   BRAIDING AND CORNROWING

As a bonus for those of you not confident in braiding or cornrowing, I've included full instructions on how to do it!

I know that for some of us, braiding and cornrowing almost seem like second nature, but there are many mums of children with kinky, curly or afro-textured hair that don't know how to braid.

Braiding textured hair is a fantastic way to keep it protected. It stops the hair from tangling, relies on minimal manipulation as it doesn't have to be done every day, and can be transformed into a variety of styles or 'braided out' out, for a more defined, curly, natural look.

CLASSIC SING BRAID / PLAIT

Also known as a plait, this is the first type of braid you need to learn before progressing on to anything else. For braids, I like to plait underhand, because it gives better tension at the base and as a result can stay in place for longer.

YOU WILL NEED:

Rat-tail comb for parting

Wide toothcomb for detangling

Butterfly clips for sectioning

HERE'S HOW YOU DO IT:

1) Part the section of hair to be braided and clip everything else away. Take 3 sections of hair in equal size.

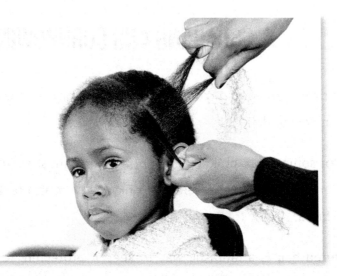

2) In one hand, hold two of the sections, one between your index and middle finger and the other between your thumb and index finger. In the other hand, hold one section between your index and middle finger.

3) The middle section will be in between your thumb and index finger. And to plait the hair, we need to use a simple right-under-middle, then left-under-middle pattern.

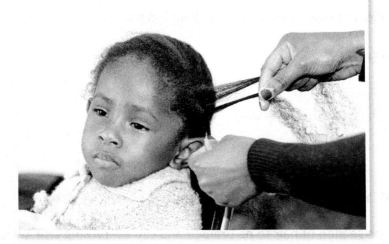

4) Take the right side section of hair and move it so it goes under the middle section and ends up in the middle.

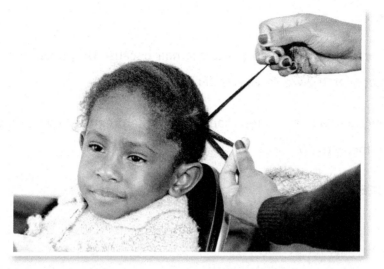

5) Then take the left side section of hair and move under the middle section so it becomes the middle section.

6) Repeat until the braid is your desired length.

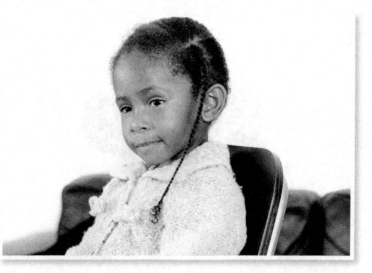

Braids are perfect for babies, toddlers and young children and can be left in the hair for ideally a week, but can also stretch to two weeks.

CORNROWS

These braids are fantastic in highly textured hair because they keep the hair protected and stay in place for 1–2 weeks as standard.

Although they seem and look more complicated than regular braids, they are not that much more difficult to do.

YOU WILL NEED:

Rat-tail comb for parting

Wide toothcomb for detangling

Butterfly clips for sectioning

1) Larger cornrows are best for learning on, so start by parting the hair from front to back. Plan your first row: part it out and clip everything else away.

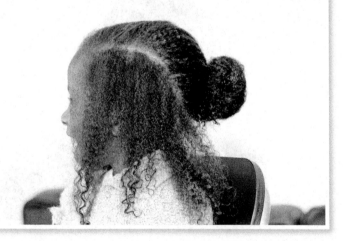

2) Make sure the hair to be cornrowed is detangled completely.

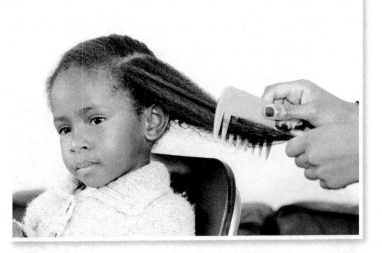

3) Position your child in front of you and, at the front of the row, start with a small section of hair divided into 3 equal-sized sections.

4) In one hand, hold 2 of the sections of hair, one in between your index finger and thumb and the other between your index and middle finger. In the other hand, hold the last section in between your thumb and middle finger.

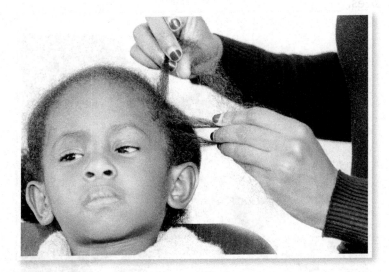

5) Start off by doing 1 rotation of a normal braid (right-under-middle, then left-under-middle pattern), but on the third rotation, as you go to grab the right section to put it in the middle, pick up some hair from underneath.

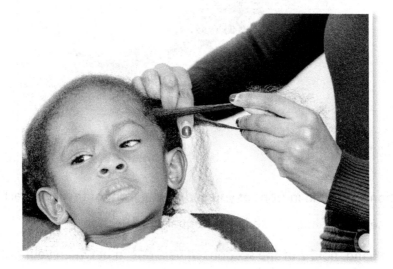

6) You only pick up when going under the middle section! And try to pick up in equal sizes.

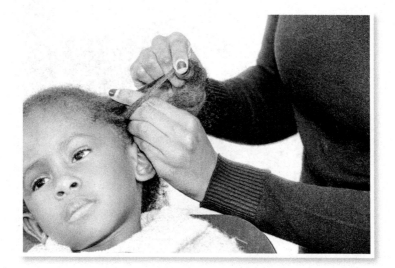

7) So as you continue doing your braid, and as you pick up hair when going under the middle section, the plait will travel backwards.

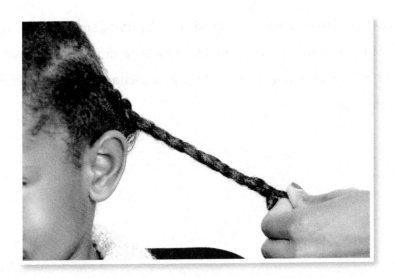

8) Continue for as far back as you want the cornrow to go.

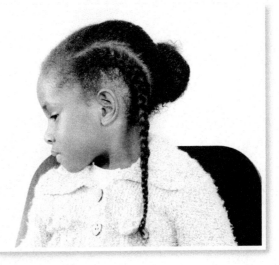

9) Part out the next row and continue.

MORE CORNROW STYLES

Mastering cornrows does take practice, and it's a good idea to get a practice head instead of experimenting on a fidgety child if you're still learning!

When you are confident enough, you can advance by trying smaller cornrows, cornrows into buns, bunches and fun styles. It's possible to create almost any style with cornrows; you just need to use your imagination. Part and section the hair carefully to create pretty much any style.

CHAPTER 23   OVERCOMING COMMON PROBLEMS AND FAQS

On your healthy hair journey with your daughter, you will have successes, but you will also encounter obstacles or setbacks. We all will. The good news is they can be overcome.

In this chapter, I will go through the top complaints I hear from mums and provide some solutions.

THE DRYNESS PROBLEM

Complaint: "My daughter's hair is just so dry"

The main problem I hear from mothers is a complaint of dryness. To them, their daughters' hair looks, feels and acts dry, and they are frustrated. No matter what they do, they can't seem to hydrate the hair properly or get it to stay hydrated for a decent amount of time.

Dry hair is dangerous because it is caused by a loss of moisture from the hair shaft, which results in inelastic hair that is prone to breakage.

POSSIBLE CAUSES

Below find a list of some factors that could be contributing to this problem.

> Using a non-water-based moisturizer

> Not following up washing with conditioning

> Not sealing moisture into the hair

> Using incorrect shampoo

> Low or high porosity hair

> Using direct heat too often

> Using a cotton pillow case or head scarf

THE SOLUTIONS

> Use a moisturizer that has water listed as the first ingredient. Or mix your own using distilled water and other ingredients of your choice. Be sure to moisturize the hair at least once a day.

> Be sure to follow up washing the hair with conditioning, to replace any moisture the shampoo may have stripped.

> Always seal the moisture into the hair with an oil or an oil followed by a cream or butter. If you are using a light oil, such as coconut oil, then try using a heavier oil such as castor oil. For dryer hair, use the LOC method, which is liquid, then oil and then a cream to really make sure the moisture doesn't escape!

> Make sure to use a mild and natural shampoo that contains no harsh surfactants. Also pre-shampoo the hair using a penetrating oil, such as coconut oil, to reduce moisture loss. For cases of drier hair, use a conditioner instead of shampoo to co-wash the hair.

> Low porosity hair has the tendency for moisture to pass easily out of the hair shaft, while high porosity has the tendency to not absorb water well. Test the hairs' porosity, and use suitable products.

> Try to limit the use of direct heat through blow-dryers and flat irons, and definitely don't use them on a regular basis. If they are used, then be sure to use a heat protectant first. Where possible, try to air-dry the hair as much as possible.

> A considerable amount of moisture will be lost to cotton sheets; to limit this, try using a satin pillow case or satin cap, as they absorb less moisture from the hair.

THE GROWTH PROBLEM

Complaint: "My daughter's hair doesn't grow"

In the absence of any medical condition, we now know that all hair grows, even if we are not seeing the length the hair is growing. This is likely not a hair growth issue; it is likely a length retention issue. This issue is very common. Thankfully, it can be overcome, and your daughter can grow long hair if you so desire.

Keep in mind that a key contributor to hair that doesn't appear to grow is what's known as 'short hair syndrome,' which is where the hair breaks abnormally just as fast as it grows.

POSSIBLE CAUSES

> Dry hair

> Brittle hair

> Wrong tools and appliances

> Incorrect hair practices

> Lack of protective styles

THE SOLUTIONS

> Dryness is a key contributor to inelasticity, which causes hair to become vulnerable to breakage. Combat this by moisturizing daily and restricting the use of heated appliances such as blow-dryers.

> Hair that has been allowed to become dry will in turn become brittle; due to in-elasticity, acts such as combing the hair will cause breakage. Make sure the hair is moisturized regularly to stave off dryness.

> Make sure to use tools that don't snag the hair, which can result in breakage. All combs should be seamless, and if a brush is used, then use a quality brush

such as a Denman brush or tangle teaser. Limit the use of heated appliances, and if they must be used, always use a heat protectant first.

> Breakage can occur when we manipulate the hair incorrectly. Make sure to use a soft hand when dealing with hair and to also always detangle or comb hair starting at the ends to limit breakage.

> Leaving the hair exposed to the elements can cause dryness and breakage. When aiming for a length goal, implement the use of protective styles to minimize breakage along the way.

THE NO EDGES PROBLEM

Complaint: *"My daughter's hair is really thin at the edges"*
This is a common complaint and one that I made myself. It can seem that the density of hair at the hairline can change. This can be attributed primarily to two factors.

POSSIBLE CAUSES

1) New hair growth – It can sometimes be difficult to tell the difference between new hair and hair breakage. But in the early years from 0–2, as the head grows new areas of hair will sprout up around the perimeter of the head.

2) Tension hair loss/breakage – This is caused by incorrect styling methods, where the hair is pulled too tightly, which results in it snapping off or being pulled out from the root.

THE SOLUTIONS

> Any new hair growth will need to be nurtured. As we primarily focus our moisturizing efforts on the mid lengths to the ends of the hair, we can sometimes forget about new growth, which can leave it vulnerable to dryness

and breakage. Instead, aim to keep the new growth just as moisturized as the ends of the hair. Using a baby brush, apply a natural moisturizer, followed by a natural oil to seal twice daily. Be gentle with this hair, and as it grows it will be long enough to incorporate in with the rest of the hair.

> The solution to tension-related hair loss or damage is simple. Apply less pressure when styling the hair and avoid tight styles! Tight styles don't make the hair grow any faster or look any better and are best avoided. Instead of corn-rowing the hair going all backwards, try putting some braids going down towards the ears in the hairline. Also stop using rubber bands when styling a child's hair, as these often cause damage. Instead, use a cotton band, a seamless band or an "ouch-less" band.

THE DRY SPOT PROBLEM

Complaint: "There's just one patch of hair that's dry"

This happens often and it happened to my daughter. She had one patch of hair in her crown that was excessively dry. When moisture was applied to it, the hair absorbed it up almost instantly and would then be dry again.

It's important we keep all the hair moisturized so it can all grow together; the problem with a dry patch is that it might fall behind if breakage occurs.

POSSIBLE CAUSES

> Rubbing

> Incorrect products

> Lack of protective styling

THE SOLUTIONS

> Rubbing is a common cause of a dry spot in a little one's hair. It occurs where the head rubs on a bed or chair and can cause dry patches. The best thing to do if this is happening with your child is to pay special attention to that area and moisturize it more often. It could be that the majority of the hair you moisturize 1–2 times a day, while a dry spot should be moisturized more frequently with heavier products to seal in the moisture.

> The aim of moisturizing hair is to keep it *all* hydrated. If you are finding that the moisturizer you are using is leaving the hair dry, it could be that you have selected a product too light for the hair as a whole. If you are using a water-based moisturizer, be sure to use one that also contains a humectant to draw moisture into the hair. Also consider using a heavier oil if you are using a light one, and finally consider using a heavy natural hair butter to seal the hair.

> The rubbing factor is mainly present in babies. Even though their hair is shorter, it's still important nonetheless to try and protect it. Good styles for this are comb twists and two-strand twists. It may be the case that you will have to redo these often if the hair is short, but do this until the hair grows long enough to stay in place.

THE TANGLING PROBLEM

Complaint: "Her hair just gets so tangled"

POSSIBLE CAUSES

> Insufficient detangling

> Wrong product usage

> Dryness

> Style kept for too long

> Washing in style more than once

SOLUTIONS

> Detangle properly and wash hair in sections if long enough. Make sure it's properly detangled prior to styling.

> Select products that offer the hair good 'slip' to minimize tangling when handling.

> Dry hair has the tendency to tangle. To combat this, keep the hair adequately moisturized consistently.

> Styles that are kept in the hair for a considerable amount of time are prone to tangling, which can be difficult to remove. Avoid this by limiting the length of time a hairstyle is in to 3 weeks at the absolute maximum. The ideal length of time we want to keep a style in is 1 week.

> If you are keeping in a style for an extended period of time (up to 3 weeks), then be sure to only wash the hair in its style once. This is because washing the hair in style more than this can cause the style to loosen and the loose parts will be prone to tangle.

THE BREAKAGE PROBLEM

Complaint: "Her hair just breaks all the time"

POSSIBLE CAUSES

> Breakage/Snapping

> Shedding

SOLUTIONS

The key to understanding this is to first ascertain if your daughter is suffering from breakage or shedding before applying a solution.

BROKEN OR SHED HAIR?

Shed hair

We learnt in Chapter 2 that the hair cycle consists of 3 distinct stages: growth phase, rest phase and shed phase. In the shed phase, hair that had previously been resting is released from the **bulb** so new hair can start to grow.

It's completely normal and is not anything to worry about. It's estimated that a human adult will shed up to 100 hairs a day.

Now, we don't have any problem with shed hairs. Issues arise when broken hairs are mistaken for shed hairs because we won't recognize them and the breakage will continue.

The difference between broken and shed hair

A shed hair will likely have a tiny white bulb at one end where the hair has been released from the follicle, whereas a broken hair won't have any bulb and may have sharp angles at its ends.

It's normal when you are washing, styling or detangling hair to see some hair in the comb, sink or your hands. But it's not normal if it's caused by breakage. To know for sure if you are dealing with hair breakage, you're going to need to investigate.

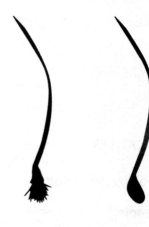

Broken Hair   *Shed* Hair

The best way to do this is to go through some of this lost hair and check the ends for a tiny white bulb; if there is a bulb, it's a shed hair, and you are okay. If not, then it's possible it could be a broken hair, which is not okay.

Broken Hair

Hair breakage can be caused by the following factors:

> **Breakage through combing**

Styling and combing the hair is a culprit when it comes to causing hair breakage. Sometimes when combing hair we can inadvertently snap it, and this has to be avoided.

> **Heavy handedness**

Another cause of breakage can be rough styling; children's hair needs a delicate touch

> **Unsuitable products**

A fine-toothed comb with teeth too close together is another cause of breakage.

SOLUTIONS FOR BREAKAGE

> Check that the hair is receiving enough moisture and is not dry.

> Limit direct heat if you are using it.

> Make sure you are staying on top of a healthy hair care regime and are following all the techniques in this book.

> Make sure you are not over-moisturizing, as this can weaken hair, and make sure the hair is being allowed to fully dry before more moisturizer is applied.

> Make sure you are using quality seamless appliances that can't snag the hair.

> Make sure you are being gentle with her hair. Heavy hands are a direct cause of breakage, so be gentle!

If you haven't already then be sure to like us on Facebook as we give out daily hair care tips there!

f LIKE US: WWW.FACEBOOK.COM/NATURALHAIRCAREFORGIRLS

CHAPTER 24 FINAL THOUGHTS

Thank you!

Well, firstly, I actually just want to thank you for taking the time to read this book, and I hope it's a helpful resource for you.

I practice what I preach, and I can testify that the techniques outlined in this book do work! Although you don't have to follow what I teach to the letter, I do hope it's at least a guiding light in your hair care journey with your daughter.

My daughter has been my inspiration for this book. Seeing how much she enjoys and loves her hair was the catalyst for me writing this book, and I want your daughter to have the same experience.

No more embarrassment, no more wishing for 'different' hair...my goal is that through this book, mothers all over the world will be able to help their daughters achieve beautiful, healthy, kinky, curly and afro hair that they absolutely love!

Lulu Pierre

CPSIA information can be obtained
at www.ICGtesting.com
Printed in the USA
LVOW04s0750210118

563322LV00003B/41/P